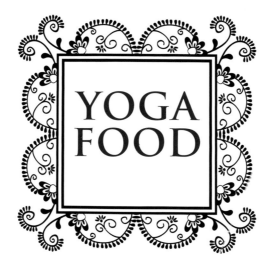

YOGA FOOD

50 Recipes for Fresh and Healthy Dishes

By Anna Gidgård and
Cecilia Davidsson

Translation by Lena Golden

Skyhorse Publishing

Thanks to Cazami and House Doctor for loaning the props.

Copyright © 2012 by Anna Gidgård and Cecilia Davidsson
Translation copyright © 2012 by Lena Golden

Originally published in Sweden by Ica Bokförlag, Forma Books AB, as *Yogamat*.

Skyhorse Publishing books may be purchased in bulk at special discounts for sales promotion, corporate gifts, fund-raising, or educational purposes. Special editions can also be created to specifications. For details, contact the Special Sales Department, Skyhorse Publishing, 307 West 36th Street, 11th Floor, New York, NY 10018 or info@skyhorsepublishing.com.

Skyhorse® and Skyhorse Publishing® are registered trademarks of Skyhorse Publishing, Inc.®, a Delaware corporation.

www.skyhorsepublishing.com

10 9 8 7 6 5 4 3 2 1

Library of Congress Cataloging-in-Publication Data is available on file.

ISBN: 978-1-62087-216-1

Printed in China

Contents

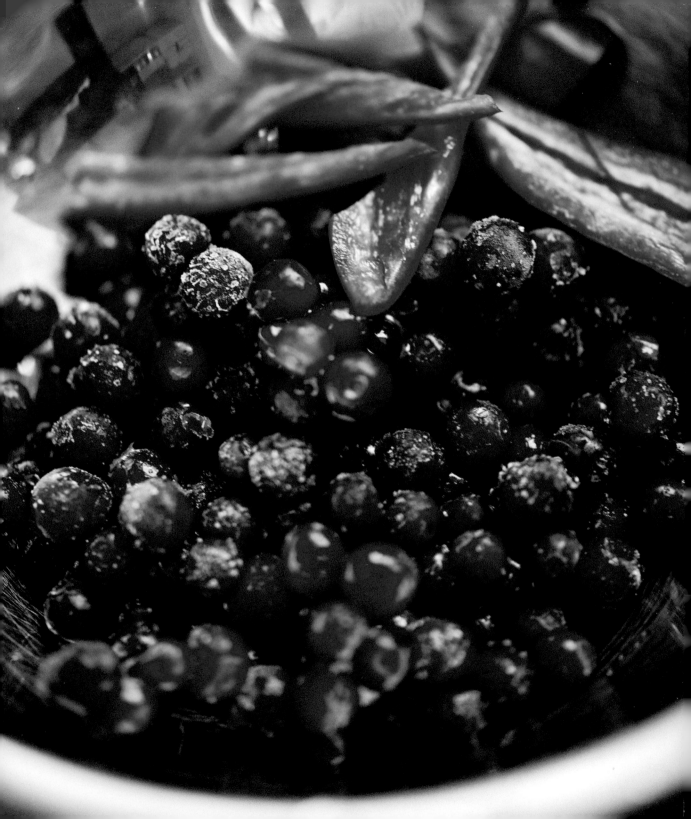

PREFACE

The idea for this book came after my first yoga retreat where Cecilia Davidsson—or Cissi, as she is called—cooked the food. For five days I was eating food that went straight into my system and did my body good. The flavors were fantastic and I felt better than ever—as well as satisfied and full. But once back home, I fell quickly back into a rut of bad eating habits.

That was when I started to think that there must be other people like me, who practice yoga or something similar that makes you aware of your body and makes you want to eat better, but who find it hard to integrate it into their everyday lives. That's when Cissi decided to write down all the wonderful dishes she created! There are power breakfasts and yoga cereal, hearty lunches, wonderful dinners, and beautiful buffets that are perfect if you want to invite your friends to something special that will make them feel good at the same time.

There are also snacks that will be great after a late yoga session, which is what you often have to do when you want to fit yoga into a typical urban or family-life schedule. Most of the ingredients can be found in any grocery store at any time, while a few need to be purchased in health food stores or in a grocery store that sells Asian specialty foods.

So now, just go for it—on the yoga mat and in the kitchen!

Anna Gidgård and Cecilia Davidsson

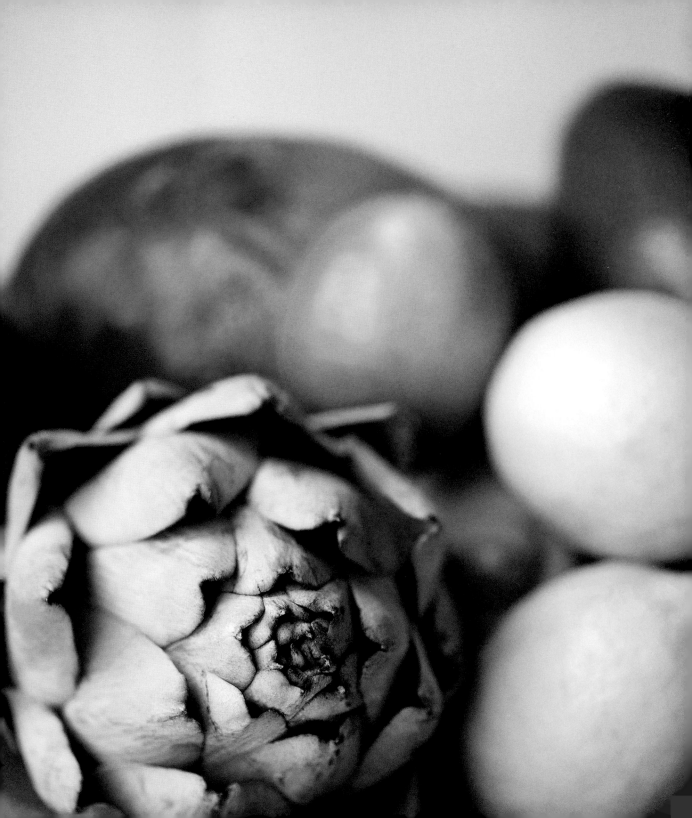

YOGA FOOD

Some things in life you cannot influence, but you can take control of and change what you eat. It is possible to reverse a downward spiral with little changes. You deserve good food!

A person who practices yoga needs to eat foods that provide energy but also create a balance of mind. Yoga can be very physical, and you will need highly nutritious food. In this book, we avoid refined products like white flour and sugar, and we also avoid milk. However, we use yogurt because it contains probiotics—good bacteria. The dishes contain a lot of different vegetables and we use many different cooking methods in order to give you a wide variety of nutrition as well as many flavors and textures. There is food that may not be heated at all, and some that may for example be steamed or roasted.

Yoga food is light, crunchy, and flavorful. Crunchy nuts and fresh vegetables provide crispness and something to chew; whole grains provide fiber and fill you up for a long time. Soy sauce, chili peppers, and fresh herbs add flavor. Sweet fruits and berries are used in desserts and baked goods to create pleasure and satisfaction.

Ayurvedic principles are the basis for yoga food. But the dishes that you enjoy and that make you feel good are individual and depend on body type. When you practice yoga and are physically active, often you will find yourself craving the foods that your body needs. Just as in the Ayurvedic teachings, there should be a balance in yoga food between raw and cooked food. It has to be easy to digest, fresh, freshly made, contain enzymes, and be full of fiber, whole grains, and good bacteria.

Choose from seasonal local produce as much as possible. Remember to eat in a calm environment and not too late. You will notice that it gets a little easier to avoid snacking and fast food if you eat foods that fill you up and make you feel satisfied.

To be completely yogic you need to eat something sweet, sour, salty, bitter, pungent, and astringent every day, but avoid alcohol and sugar as much as possible, and completely get rid of caffeine and tobacco.

Avoid eating too heavy a meal at night. This will not only help you sleep better, but also give you a sense of lightness when doing yoga in the morning. Try to eat some raw food with all meals. Leafy greens and sprouts contain chlorophyll, enzymes, and minerals—things that strengthen the body.

Yoga itself promotes a regular stomach, but this kind of food helps even more. Good-quality food that makes you feel good is often very simple. A lot of times you can just take a vegetable, shred it, drizzle olive oil on it, sprinkle it with lemon, salt, and pepper, and you have a delicious meal!

It's wonderful to first do yoga and then eat a meal that is pure, organic, and packed with nutrition. It's like a double dose of wellness.

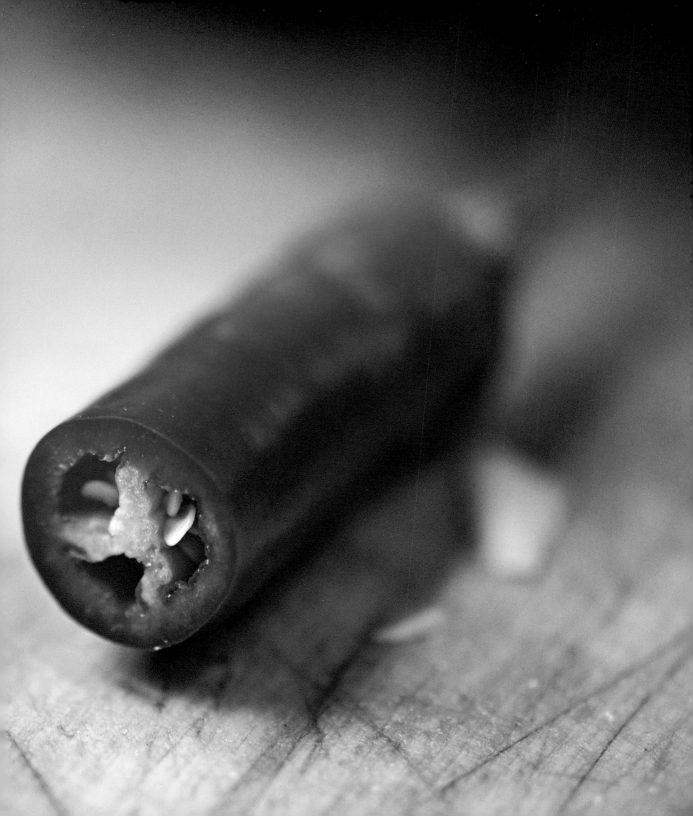

INGREDIENTS

Here are some of the foods that we think are particularly exciting. Some are naturally free from gluten while others are rich in antioxidants and have anti-inflammatory properties. What they all have in common is that they are good for both body and soul and therefore work well as yoga food.

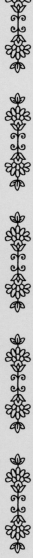

AGAVE NECTAR

Agave nectar is a sweet syrup derived from agave. It does not spike blood sugar as fast as sugar, but it's still a carbohydrate that should be used in moderation.

ALMONDS

Almonds are rich in vitamin E and tryptophan, an amino acid. They have a large amount of monounsaturated fat, and also a lot of protein. Almonds, like many nuts and seeds, contain antioxidants.

AMARANTH

Amaranth is a seed that is naturally gluten-free and contains more protein and calcium than milk. It is sold as small seeds or in ground powder form. Cook the whole seeds with rice or quinoa, add a few tbsp of amaranth flour to a soup as a thickener, use it for hot cereal, or stir cooked seeds into bread dough. Amaranth is related to spinach and quinoa.

BLUEBERRIES

Blueberries are rich in vitamins C and A, as well as manganese. They have a positive effect on the stomach and are super antioxidant berries. Use fresh, frozen, or dried berries. There are also blueberries in powder form. Blueberries help the body create the hormone dopamine, which is necessary for well-being, memory, and concentration.

CARROTS

Carrots are rich in vitamin A, carotenoids, B vitamins, phosphorus, iodine, and calcium, and are good for night vision, the skin, the lungs, the liver, and the pancreas. Nowadays, we can get heirloom carrots in colors like yellow, red, and purple.

CASHEWS

Cashews have a neutral, sweet taste and contain healthy fats, minerals, and some protein. You can roast them and sprinkle them over a dish or eat them as snacks. I use them in soups for creaminess, and for lemon curd, blended as a substitute for heavy cream. Another good idea is to mix them with raw vegetables, onion, and lemon juice, and spice the mixture up with tamari and pepper to make a good, wholesome dip.

CHIA SEEDS

Chia seeds are similar to flaxseed but are more nutritious. Chia seeds are rich in protein, fiber, omega-3, and various antioxidants. These make chia seeds more long-lasting than flaxseed, which can easily go rancid after having been milled. You could definitely put the seeds in water and then drink the gelatinous liquid that it makes. I put my seeds in smoothies, pancake batter, super-food cakes, hot cereal, and muesli. If you can't get chia seeds, you can substitute flaxseed.

CHLORELLA

Chlorella is a sweet algae. It is nutritious and chock full of chlorophyll. You can use chlorella as a nutrition boost in your smoothie or drink iced herbal tea with it. It is sold in health food stores and online. If you have no access to chlorella, you can also use spirulina, a green powder that is sold in different varieties and products, or use flaxseed.

COCONUT OIL

Organic unrefined coconut oil has many health benefits. One is that it contains lauric acid,

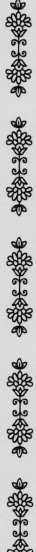

which is also found in breast milk. It enhances brain function and the immune system. Unrefined coconut oil is free of trans fats. You can fry with it, bake with it, and mix it into smoothies. If you replace the fat in pie dough with coconut oil, you can use 25 percent less fat. You can also buy flavorless coconut oil.

GINGER

Ginger has a warming effect, stimulates digestion, and helps circulation. Ginger is effective for colds, fever, and nausea. More ginger to the people!

ROSE HIPS

Rose hips are a good source of vitamin C and contain antioxidants, beta-carotene, and various minerals. They have anti-inflammatory effects and may work against arthritis.

SESAME OIL

Cold-pressed sesame oil is used as regular oil. You cannot use it in place of the strongly sesame-flavored toasted sesame oil used in cuisines such as Thai, but you may substitute it for olive oil.

TOFU AND TEMPEH

Tofu is made from soybeans. It supports the intestines and lungs and is especially good for people who feel warm or have high blood pressure. Tofu is rich in protein and is available in a few different consistencies. Firm tofu can be marinated with spices, herbs, tamari, garlic, ginger, and lemon with great results.

Another favorite is tempeh, made from fermented soybeans. It is common in Indonesian cooking. It has a denser consistency than tofu, and it is a good alternative to meat in terms of protein and nutrition. It is a bit harder to come by but is sold in health food stores and Asian supermarkets. You can fry it, roast it, or steam it.

FAVORITES IN THE KITCHEN

In the pantry: miso, tamari, agave nectar, maple syrup, apple cider vinegar, chipotle Tabasco, olive oil, coconut oil, seaweed, beans, lentils, dried fruit, cocoa, coconut, vanilla, nuts, seeds, licorice, brown rice, quinoa, amaranth, chia seeds, buckwheat . . .

The spice rack: among others, cumin, fennel, coriander, cinnamon, and cardamom.

In the refrigerator: eggs, cheese, and yogurt . . .

Almost every day I eat: lemon, ginger, garlic, chili pepper, avocado, fresh fruit and vegetables, mushrooms, fresh herbs . . .

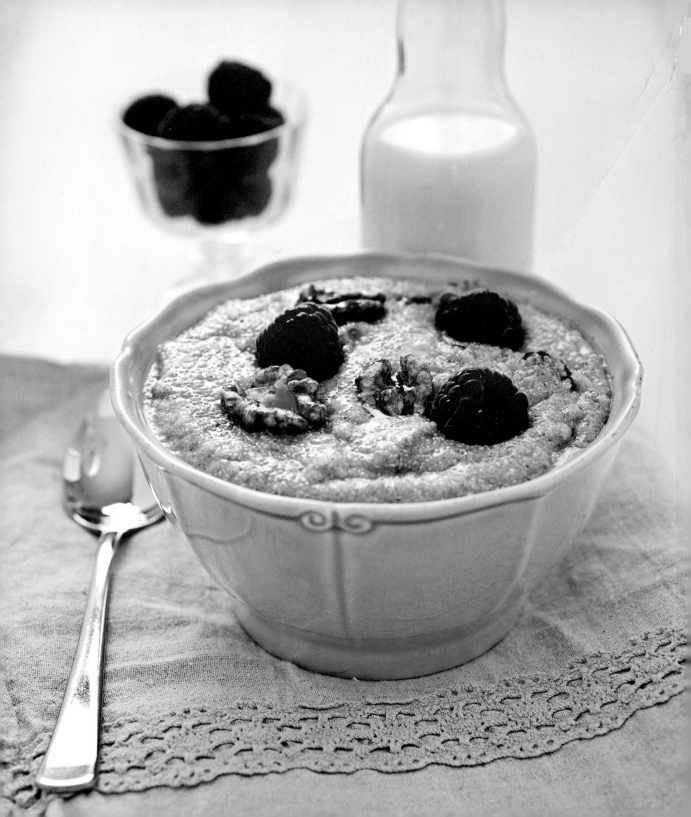

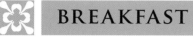

Hot Amaranth Cereal with Vanilla

Mild, creamy, and super healthy! If you have any left over, you can heat it up another day.

4 servings
1 scant cup (200 ml) amaranth or millet
1/2 tsp vanilla
salt
1 tbsp butter
milk, nuts, fruits, and berries for serving

DIRECTIONS:

1. The night before: Place amaranth in a saucepan and add 1 3/4 cups (400 ml) water. Leave overnight.
2. The next morning: Add 1/4 cup (50 ml) water, vanilla, and a pinch of salt. Bring to boil and let the cereal simmer for about 10 minutes on low heat. Stir in the butter.
3. Serve with milk, chopped nuts, fruits, and berries.

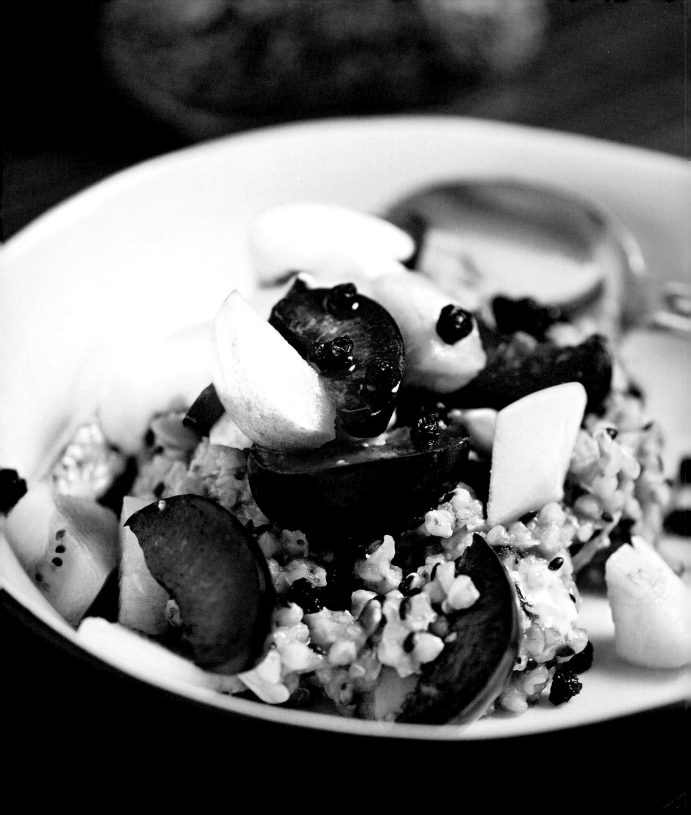

Yoga Cereal

This is a classic at every yoga retreat where I have made the food. One time, everybody wanted hot buckwheat cereal, but I noticed that many people had a blood-sugar drop after breakfast, so I boosted it with quinoa and seeds. It feels good and fills you up! I serve the porridge with additions such as fresh fruit, dried blueberries, apple compote, cinnamon, cardamom, coconut, or nuts.

4 servings

1 scant cup (200 ml) mixed grains, recipe to
   follow
2 tbsp dried fruit, such as raisins, finely chopped
   apricots, or goji berries
sea salt
butter or coconut oil

DIRECTIONS:

1. The night before: Combine mixed grains
   with 2 cups (500 ml) water in a saucepan.
   Bring to a boil and drain off the water. Add
   1 3/4 cups (400 ml) of cold water. Leave out
   till next morning.
2. In the morning: Add 1 scant cup (200 ml)
   water, 2 tbsp dried fruit, and 1/4 tsp sea salt
   to the grain mixture. Bring to a boil

and let simmer over low heat for 5–10
   minutes until it reaches the desired consistency. Stir in a knob of butter or coconut oil.
3. Serve with various toppings and yogurt or
   milk to taste.

Grain Mix for Yoga Cereal

Make a big batch and leave the jar of ready-mixed grains out on your counter to make it easier to remember to soak for the next morning.

3 1/2 cups (800 ml) whole buckwheat
1 scant cup (200 ml) quinoa or millet
1/2 cup (100 ml) flaxseed
1/2 cup (100 ml) sunflower seeds
1/2 cup (100 ml) pumpkin seeds

DIRECTIONS:
1. Put all ingredients in a jar and shake.

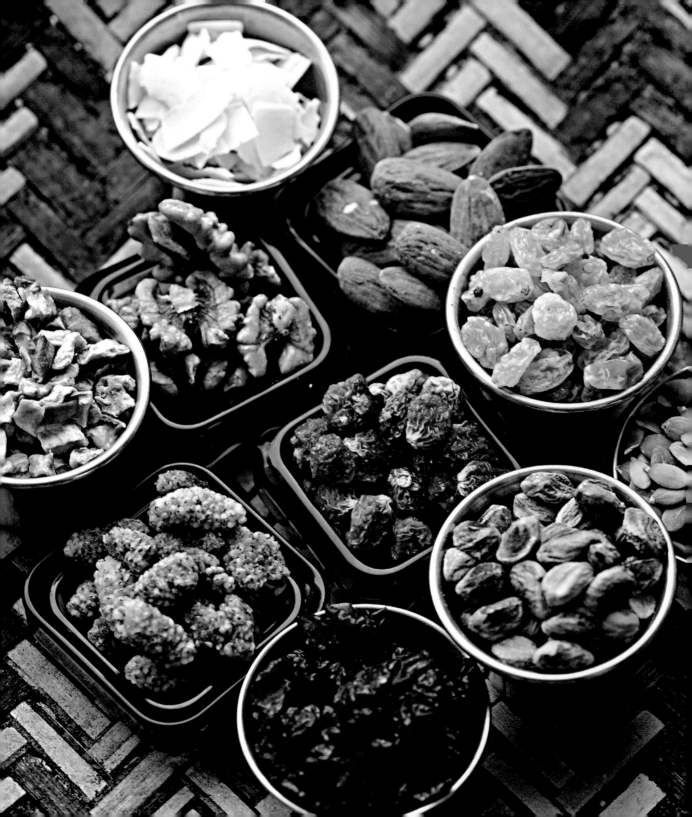

Jazz Up Your Cereal!

Dried berries, raisins, goji berries, pieces of apple, mulberries, and black and golden raisins give wonderfully tangy sweetness. Shredded toasted coconut lends a luxurious touch. Pistachios, almonds, and pumpkin seeds give cereal a crunch!

Yoga spices (see below) are something that are really good to have in a little jar and sprinkle over your cereal to spice up the taste of your breakfast. The spices can also be used in smoothies, in desserts with dried fruit and nuts, and in cake batter!

Blueberry Spice

1/2 cup (100 ml) dried blueberry powder
1 scant cup (200 ml) shredded coconut
1 tbsp ground cardamom
1 tsp ground vanilla bean or the seeds of
   1 vanilla bean

DIRECTIONS:
1. Place all ingredients in a blender and blend until fine. Store in a jar with a lid and use as a topping on oatmeal and yogurt.

Rosehip Spice

1/2 cup (100 ml) rosehip powder
1 scant cup (200 ml) shredded coconut
1 tbsp cinnamon
1/2 tbsp ground cardamom
1 tsp ground ginger
1 pinch of nutmeg

DIRECTIONS:
1. Place all ingredients in a blender and blend until fine. Keep in a jar with a lid and use as a topping on oatmeal and yogurt.

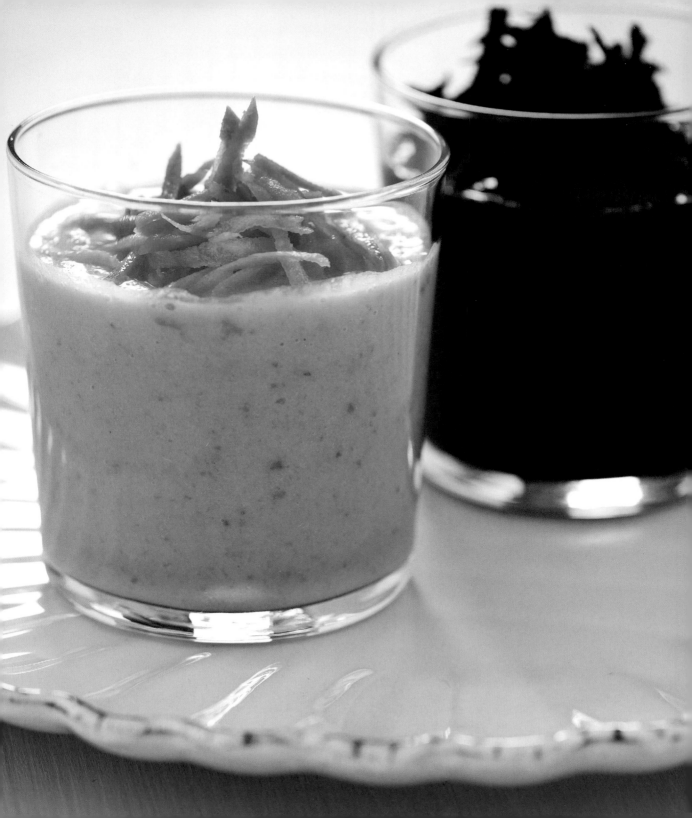

Carrot Smoothie with Apple and Coconut

This has a fresh flavor and is smooth because of the coconut milk. Rich in fiber, and filling!

2 servings
1 orange
1 apple
2 carrots
1 banana
1/2 cup (100 ml) coconut milk
1/2 cup (100 ml) apple juice (preferably fresh juice of the apple)

DIRECTIONS:
1. Squeeze the orange. Coarsely grate the apple and carrot (peel if needed). Break the banana into pieces.
2. Mix everything with coconut milk and apple juice.

To the left, Carrot Smoothie with Apple and Coconut
To the right, Beet and Raspberry Smoothie with a Boost
(recipe on following page).

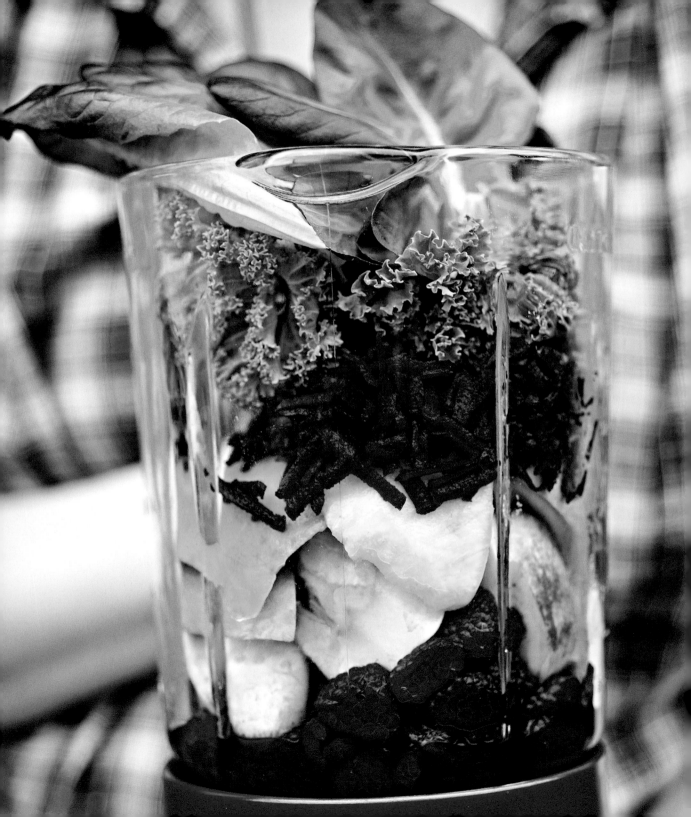

Beet and Raspberry Smoothie with a Boost

Leafy greens are amazingly useful. If you find it difficult to eat enough, you can sneak them in by drinking them in tangy smoothies filled to the brim with minerals, enzymes, antioxidants, vitamins, and chlorophyll. Drink one of these a day and see what it does to your body.

1–2 servings
1 beet
1/4 pineapple
1/2 avocado
a few broccoli florets
1/2 cup (100 ml) raspberries
3 large lettuce leaves, such as lollo rosso, or 2 handfuls of arugula, or a bunch of parsley
1/2 cup (100 ml) apple juice

DIRECTIONS:
1. Peel and grate the beet coarsely. Cut the pineapple into chunks. Scoop out the avocado flesh. Cut the broccoli into pieces.
2. Blend all ingredients together for a smooth, healthy drink.

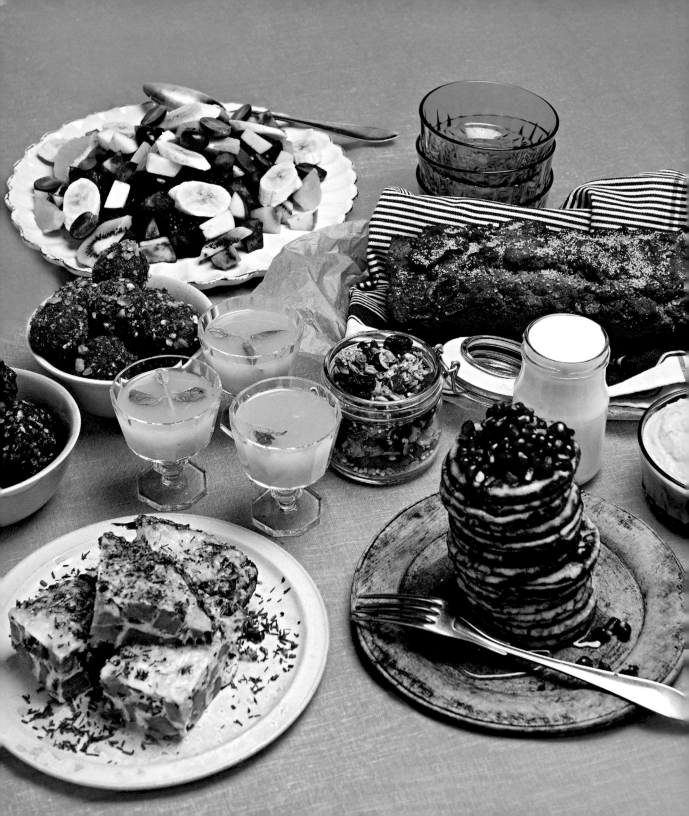

YOGA BRUNCH

The dishes for yoga brunch work really well together, but you can obviously serve these dishes individually as well. You could swap your usual weekend breakfast for the pancakes or serve the sweet potato tortilla for lunch with a simple salad.

Lemon Curd

1 1/2 cups (300 ml) cashews
3/4 cup (150 ml) agave nectar
juice and finely grated zest of 3 lemons
optional: coarse sea salt

DIRECTIONS:

1. Grind cashew nuts, agave nectar, and lemon juice in a blender until smooth. Add the finely grated lemon zest to taste, and if needed add a pinch of sea salt.

Apple Juice with Orange and Mint

A nice little thirst quencher and vitamin boost.

4 small servings
6 apples
3 oranges
mint or lemon balm for garnish

DIRECTIONS:

1. Run the apples through a juice extractor. Squeeze the oranges.
2. Mix juices and garnish with mint or lemon balm.

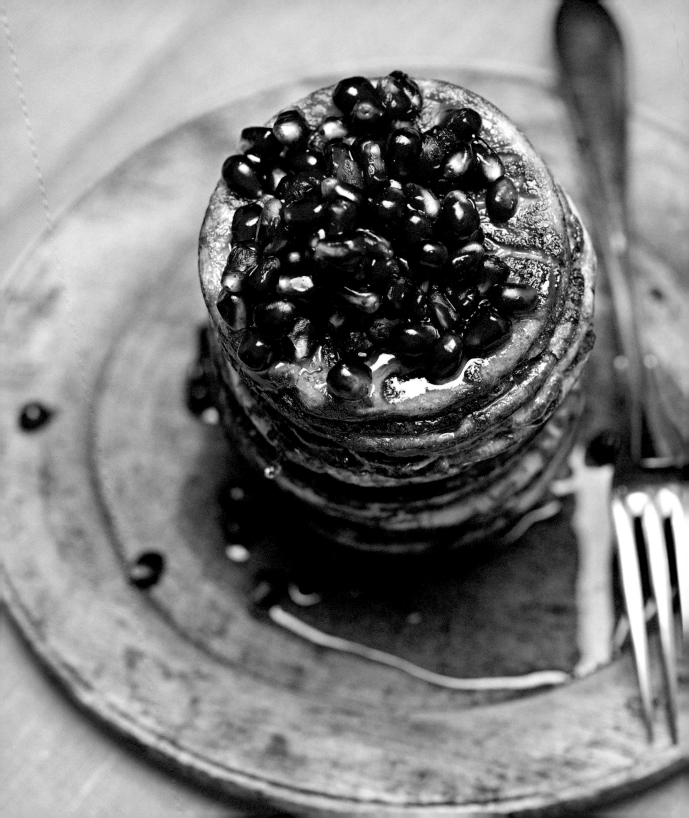

Coconut Pancakes

These pancakes are great, with a sweet coconut flavor. They contain rice flour and are naturally gluten-free. They are filling, since they contain the healthy coconut fat from coconut oil, and you can make them as crepes with a side of vegetables.

About 25 pancakes

1 scant cup (200 ml) rice flour

2 pinches sea salt

3 eggs

1 1/4 cup (300 ml) coconut milk

2 tbsp coconut oil for frying

Serve with: agave nectar or maple syrup, and pomegranate seeds

DIRECTIONS:

1. Whisk all ingredients together into a batter. Let rest for 15 minutes.

2. Fry the pancakes in coconut oil in a crepe pan over medium-high heat.

3. Drizzle pancakes with agave nectar or maple syrup and top with pomegranate seeds.

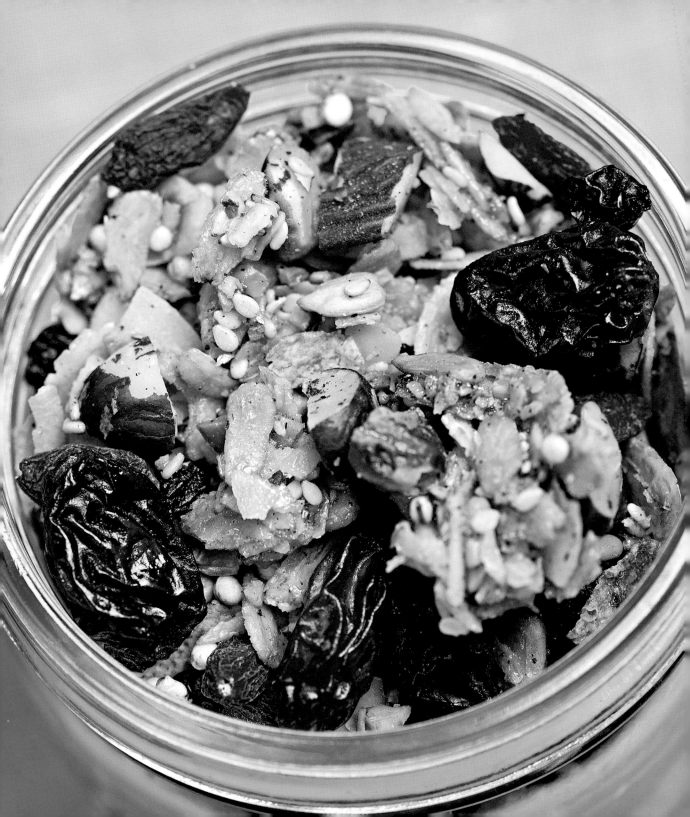

Yummy Muesli

This is a crunchy muesli that contains everything your body needs. Sprinkle it over a creamy yogurt and seasonal fruit salad.

1/2 cup (100 ml) almonds

3 cups (700 ml) rolled spelt

1 scant cup (200 ml) shredded coconut

1/2 cup (100 ml) sunflower seeds

1/2 cup (100 ml) pumpkin seeds

1/2 cup (100 ml) hazelnuts

1/4 cup (50 ml) sesame seeds

3 tbsp coconut oil

1/4 cup (50 ml) apple juice, preferably cider

1/4 cup (50 ml) rice syrup or maple syrup

1 tsp ground vanilla bean

1/2 cup (100 ml) quinoa puffs (like puffed rice)

1 scant cup (200 ml) spelt flakes (a healthy variation of corn flakes)

1 1/2 cups (300 ml) dried fruits (raisins, goji berries, blueberries, cranberries, and currants)

DIRECTIONS:

1. Set the oven to 300°F (150°C). Line a cookie sheet with edges with parchment paper.
2. Chop the almonds coarsely. Mix them together with the rolled spelt, coconut, sunflower seeds, pumpkin seeds, hazelnuts, and sesame seeds in a large mixing bowl.
3. Melt the coconut oil in a saucepan and pour it over the dry mixture along with apple juice, rice syrup, and ground vanilla bean. Mix well, preferably with your hands.
4. Spread it on the cookie sheet and roast for about 30 minutes until the muesli has a light-brown color and a lovely aroma fills the kitchen.
5. Let the muesli cool off and add puffed quinoa, spelt flakes, and dried berries.
6. Store the muesli in a jar with a lid.

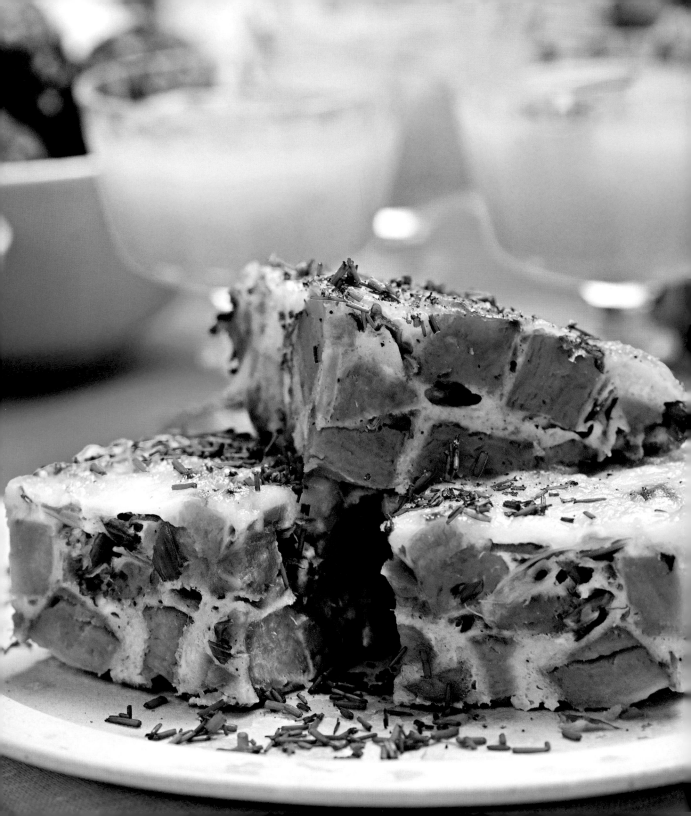

Sweet Potato Frittata

Wholesome and tasty, with a lovely juicy texture. Along with a simple green salad, it also makes for a good lunch or dinner.

For 4 people (8 buffet servings)

1 lb (500 g) sweet potatoes

1/3 leek (use the entire leek, both white and green parts)

2 cloves garlic

3/8 cup (75 ml) coconut oil

sea salt and black pepper

5 eggs

3 1/2 oz (100 g) grated cheese

1 bunch chives for garnish

DIRECTIONS:

1. Preheat the oven to 400°F (200°C). Peel sweet potatoes and cut into cubes. Slice leeks. Peel and mince the garlic.

2. Heat an oven-safe pan. Add half the coconut oil and the cubed sweet potatoes. Fry over medium heat until softened and browned slightly and put them on a plate.

3. Heat the remaining coconut oil and fry the leeks and garlic over medium heat. Put the sweet potatoes back in and season with about 1 tsp salt and 1/2 tsp pepper.

4. Beat the eggs lightly. Pour them over the sweet potatoes and onions. Sprinkle with cheese and place the pan in the oven for 10–15 minutes.

5. Slide out the frittata onto a plate and sprinkle with chopped chives. Cut the frittata up into squares if you serve it for a buffet.

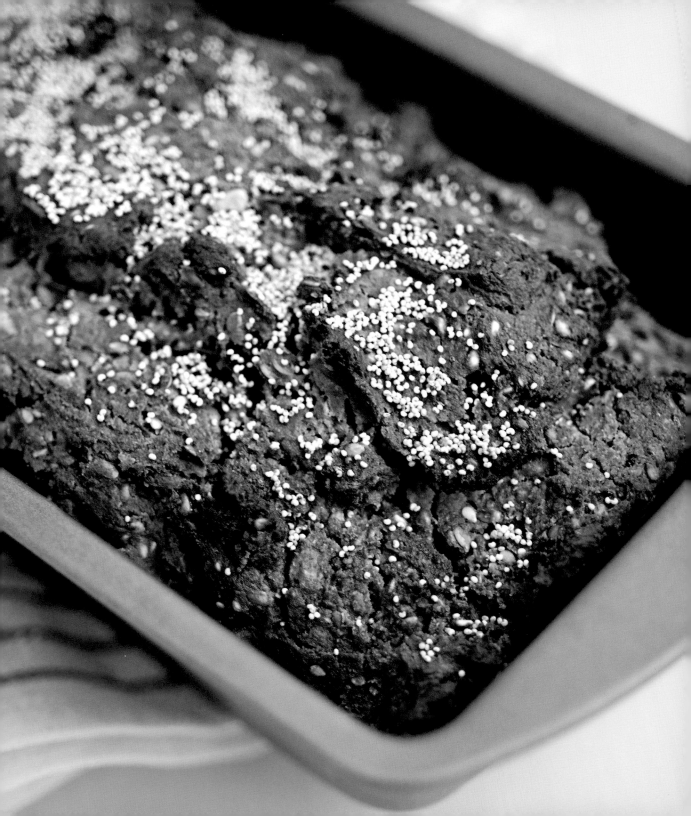

Yogi Bread

Good with soup or for breakfast. Make
sandwiches with it and it will be the perfect
late-night snack, or have it after a late yoga
class. It is gluten-free, too!

About 40 small rolls or 2 large loaves

1 3/4 oz (50 g) fresh yeast

2 tsp honey

2 1/2 cups (600 ml) water

1 3/4 cups (400 ml) millet flakes

1 1/2 cups (300 ml) buckwheat flakes
   or rice flakes

3/4 cup (150 ml) finely chopped dried apricots

1 1/2 lbs (600 g) cold cooked sweet potatoes
   (about 2 sweet potatoes)

2 cups (500 ml) water

1 3/4 cups (400 ml) sunflower seeds

1 scant cup (200 ml) flaxseed

3/4 cup (150 ml) sesame seeds

2 cups (500 ml) buckwheat flour

2 1/2 cups (600 ml) brown rice flour or
   corn flour

1–2 tsp ground fennel seeds

2 tsp sea salt

3 tbsp olive oil

coconut oil or olive oil to grease the pans

DIRECTIONS:

1. Crumble the yeast and stir in honey and
   water. Add the millet and buckwheat flakes.
   Allow to stand for about 1 hour at room
   temperature in a plastic bowl.

2. Put everything in a stand mixer and add all
   other ingredients (mash sweet potato first).
   Mix for about 10 minutes on medium speed.

3. Preheat the oven to 200°F (100°C). Spoon
   out the batter onto a cookie sheet or into two
   loaf pans greased with coconut oil. Bake rolls
   for about 40 minutes and loaves for 50
   minutes. Brush loaves with oil. Then raise
   the oven temperature to 350°F (175°C) and
   bake for another 40 minutes.

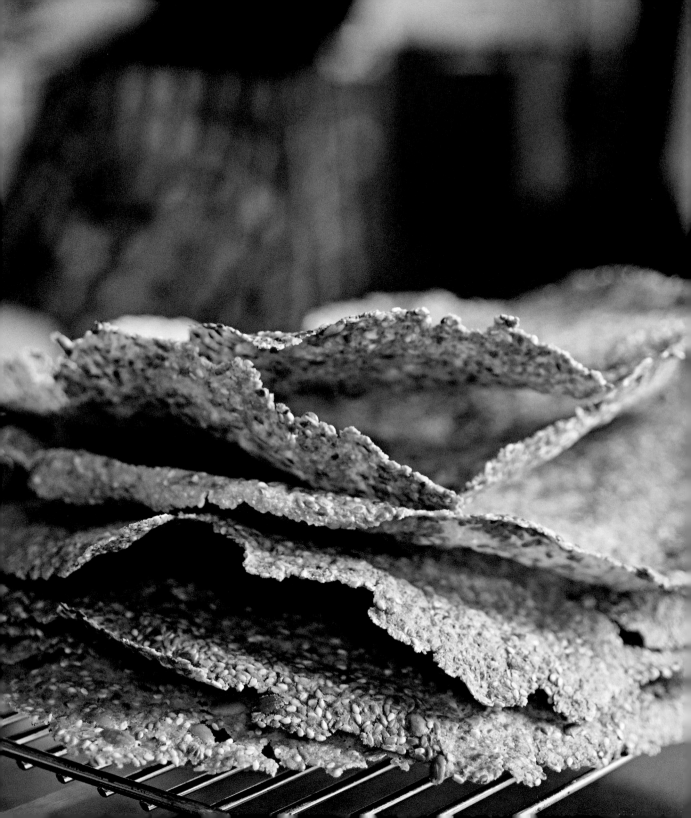

Millet Crisp Bread

Millet crisp bread is naturally gluten-free, crunchy, and good for breakfast or with dinner.

4 1/4 cups (1,000 ml) water
1/2 cup (100 ml) millet
1/2 cup (100 ml) quinoa
1 scant cup (200 ml) rice flour
1/2 cup (100 ml) sesame seeds
1/2 cup (100 ml) flaxseed
1/4 cup (50 ml) pumpkin seeds
1/2 cup (100 ml) shredded coconut
2 tbsp oil
1/2 tbsp herbal salt

DIRECTIONS:

1. Preheat the oven to 350°F (175°C). Cook water, millet, and quinoa for 15 minutes.

2. Mix in rice flour, sesame seeds, flaxseed, pumpkin seeds, coconut, oil, and herbal salt.

3. Stir into a loose dough. Roll out into thin cakes between parchment paper, place breads on cookie sheets, and bake for 35–50 minutes in the middle of the oven. You can bake two sheets at a time if you have a convection oven.

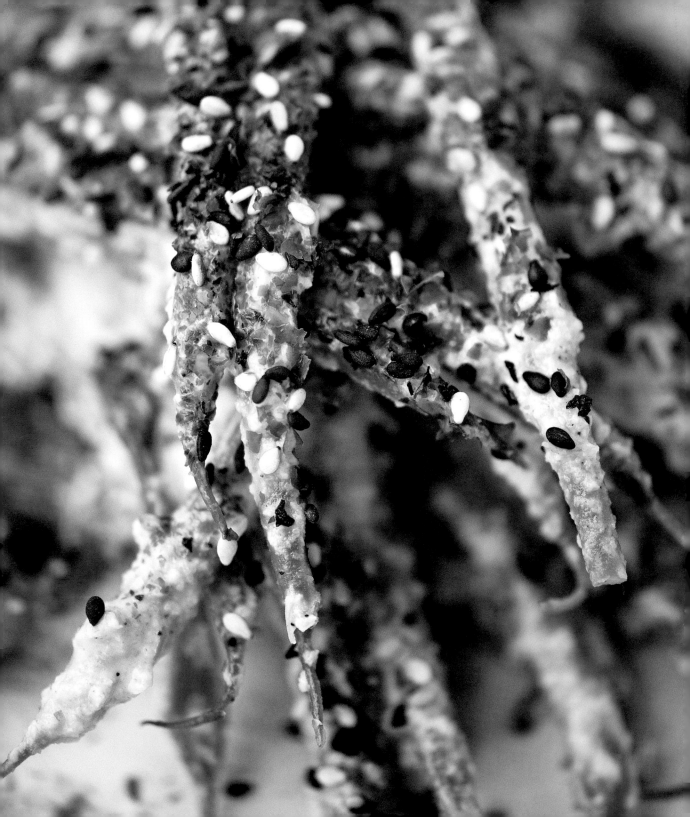

Fresh Tahini-Marinated Beans

Fresh beans are so good, you can have them as snacks! Many kids love beans. Tahini contains calcium and magnesium from sesame seeds, and beans provide both protein and fiber.

1 heaping pound (500 g) of wax beans or green beans
2 tbsp tahini
1 clove garlic
3 tbsp olive oil
1 celery stalk
1 tsp herbal salt
juice of 1/2 lemon (finely grated zest optional)
sesame seeds to sprinkle on top

DIRECTIONS:

1. Steam the beans. They should still have a crunch to them. Rinse in cold water and drain.
2. Mix tahini, grated garlic, olive oil, coarsely cut celery, herbal salt, and lemon juice into a smooth dressing.
3. Mix the dressing with the beans and allow to cool before serving. Sprinkle with sesame seeds when you are ready to serve.

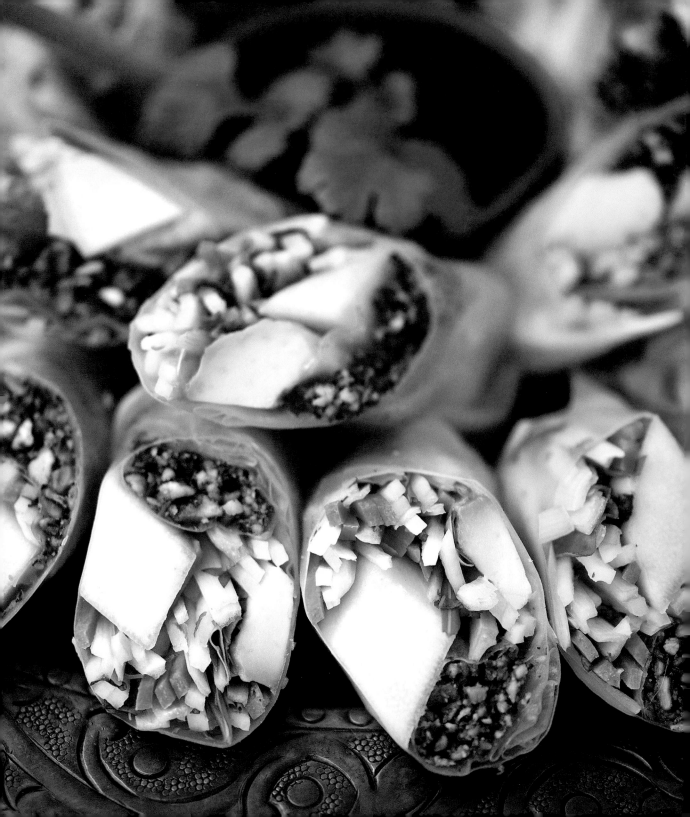

Fresh Rice Paper Rolls with Almonds

Super food with super flavor and a crunchy consistency. Perfect for a buffet!

40 pieces
20 large round sheets of rice paper
1 scant cup (200 ml) almonds
2 tbsp olive oil (or cold-pressed sesame oil)
1/2 tsp sea salt
1/2 bunch cilantro
1 carrot
1 kohlrabi
1 avocado
1 mango
1/3 leek
1/2 bunch of mint
1 1/3 oz (50 g) leafy greens, e.g. arugula, Swiss chard, mizuna, or spinach leaves

DIPPING SAUCE:
1/4 cup (50 ml) tamari
2 tsp lemon juice
2 dried apricots
1 clove garlic
3/4 inch (2 cm) ginger

DIRECTIONS:
1. Preheat the oven to 300°F (150°C). Toast the almonds in the oven for about 20 minutes. Allow to cool.
2. Mix almonds with olive oil (or sesame oil), sea salt, and cilantro.
3. Peel and julienne carrots and kohlrabi. Cut the avocado and mango into small pieces. Chop the leeks finely. Place all vegetables in a bowl along with mint and leafy greens.
4. Mix tamari, lemon juice, chopped apricots, garlic, and coarsely grated ginger with an immersion blender to form a dip. Dilute with water to loosen the consistency.
5. Dampen a kitchen towel and place it on the kitchen counter. Place a cutting board next to it. Boil water and pour it into a frying pan that you place next to the cutting board. Set the nut mix and vegetable bowl next to it.
6. Soak pieces of rice paper, place them on the towel, add some almond mixture and vegetables, and fold up into rolls according to the instructions on the package.
7. Place rolls on cutting board for now. Cut them diagonally and arrange on a serving plate. Serve with dip.

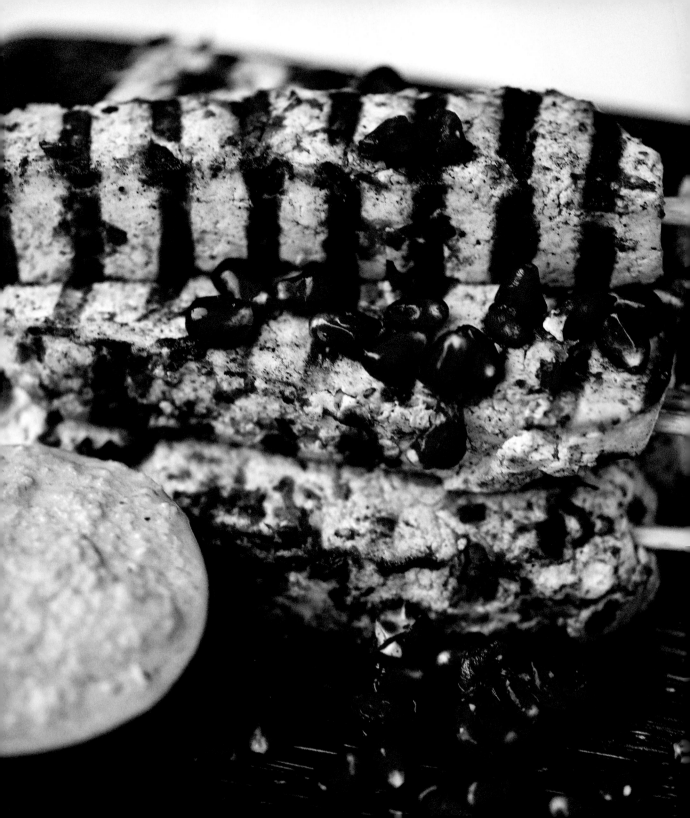

Spicy Tofu Skewers with Peanut Apple Dip

Tofu is made from soybeans. Choose organic tofu to avoid genetically modified food. Since the tofu in itself has a neutral flavor, it's suitable to be put in a marinade before cooking.

8 buffet servings
1 chili pepper
1 tbsp grated ginger
juice and finely grated peel of 1 lime
1 tsp toasted sesame oil
3 tbsp olive oil
1 tbsp miso or tamari
10 1/2 oz (300 g) tofu
pomegranate seeds for garnish

DIRECTIONS:

1. Chop chili pepper and mix with the rest of the marinade ingredients. Cut the tofu into long pieces and leave it in the marinade a few hours, preferably 24 hours.

2. Put the tofu on a skewer. Heat olive oil in a pan and fry the tofu golden-brown on each side. Pour the remaining marinade on top at the end. Serve with Peanut Apple Dip.

PEANUT APPLE DIP

A fresh nutty dip that's good for all the spicy dishes that need a little sauce.

1/2 yellow onion
1 apple
3 tbsp peanut butter
2 tbsp soy sauce
1 tbsp apple cider vinegar
2 tbsp water
1/2 tsp Tabasco sauce

DIRECTIONS:

1. Peel and cut onion into pieces. Peel, core, and cut apple into pieces.

2. Put all ingredients in a blender and blend to form a smooth dip.

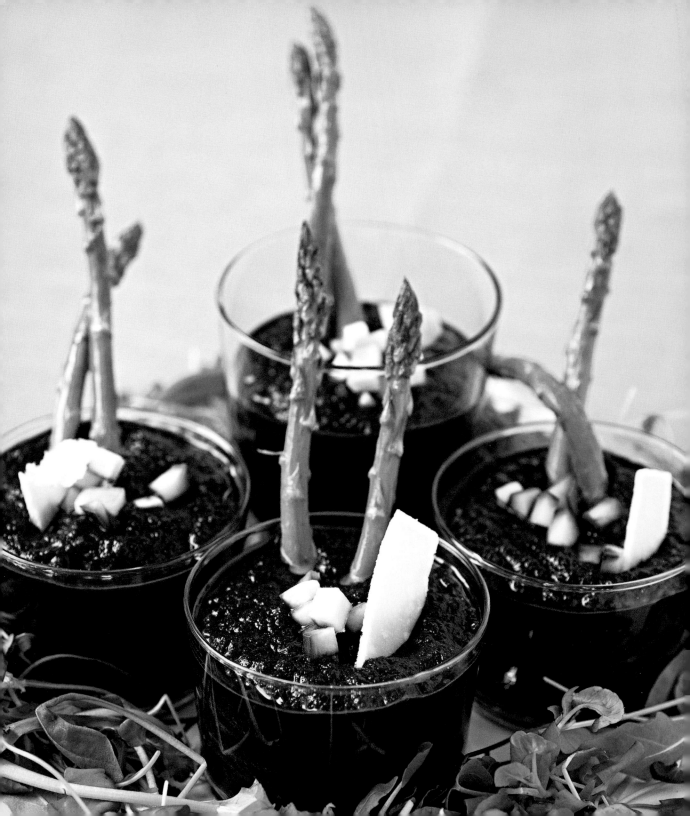

Red Beet Gazpacho

This soup is as beautiful as it is good! Beets are good for the blood, the heart, and circulation. They are at their best from harvest time in June to December.

6–8 smaller portions
5 red beets
1/2 red onion
1/2 red chili pepper
1 yellow bell pepper
1 clove garlic
1 avocado
juice of 1 lemon
1 scant cup (200 ml) water
1/2 tbsp vegetable bouillon cubes
4 ice cubes

Topping: finely diced cucumber, 1 bunch of fried asparagus, and Parmesan.

DIRECTIONS:
1. Peel and grate beets coarsely. Peel and roughly chop the onion. Coarsely chop the chili pepper and garlic. Add beets, red onion, avocado, chili pepper, bell pepper, garlic, lemon juice, water, and bouillon cube in a blender. Add ice cubes.
2. Blend until a smooth consistency. Prepare 6–8 smaller glasses. Season to taste and serve the soup in the glasses. Top with cucumber, asparagus, and Parmesan.

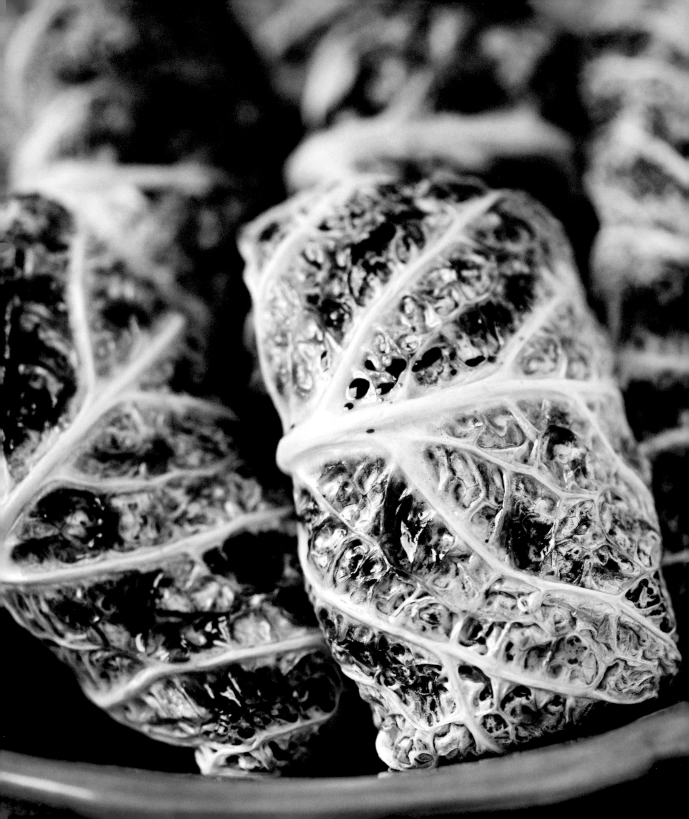

Swiss Chard Rolls

A classic for a buffet, but just as good as a hot dish served with quinoa and yogurt sauce or vegetable dip. This dish is easily varied according to season and taste. In spring, for example, fill the rolls with fresh cabbage, asparagus, fresh garlic, green peas, mint, and parsley.

Approximately 25 pieces
25 Swiss chard leaves or Savoy cabbage leaves
1 onion
1 piece of ginger
2 celery stalks
1/4 red cabbage
1 scant cup (200 ml) corn kernels
juice and grated zest of 1/2 lemon
2 tbsp tamari
1/2 cup (100 ml) grated Parmesan cheese
1/2 cup (100 ml) raisins
1/4 cup (50 ml) capers
2 tbsp finely chopped dill
sea salt and black pepper
optional: 1 egg
olive oil for brushing

DIRECTIONS:

1. Cut the stems off the chard. Put the leaves aside and save the stems as well.
2. Peel and finely chop the onion and ginger. Chop celery and chard stalks finely.
3. Fry onions and ginger in olive oil. Stir in celery and chard stalks. Cook for a few minutes and add shredded cabbage and corn kernels.
4. Stir occasionally until the cabbage has softened. Add lemon juice and tamari. Let cool.
5. Stir in the Parmesan cheese, raisins, capers, and dill. Season with salt and pepper. Add 1 egg to bind more firmly.
6. Preheat the oven to 400°F (200°C). Spread a Swiss chard leaf on a cutting board. Add about 2 tbsp of the filling and roll up the sheet starting from the longer side, and then fold the sides before you roll up the leaf completely. Secure with a toothpick if the rolls tend to open up.
7. Place the chard rolls on a cookie sheet lined with parchment paper. Brush the rolls with olive oil. Cook in the oven for about 25 minutes.
8. Serve the chard rolls with a crisp salad and a yummy sauce.

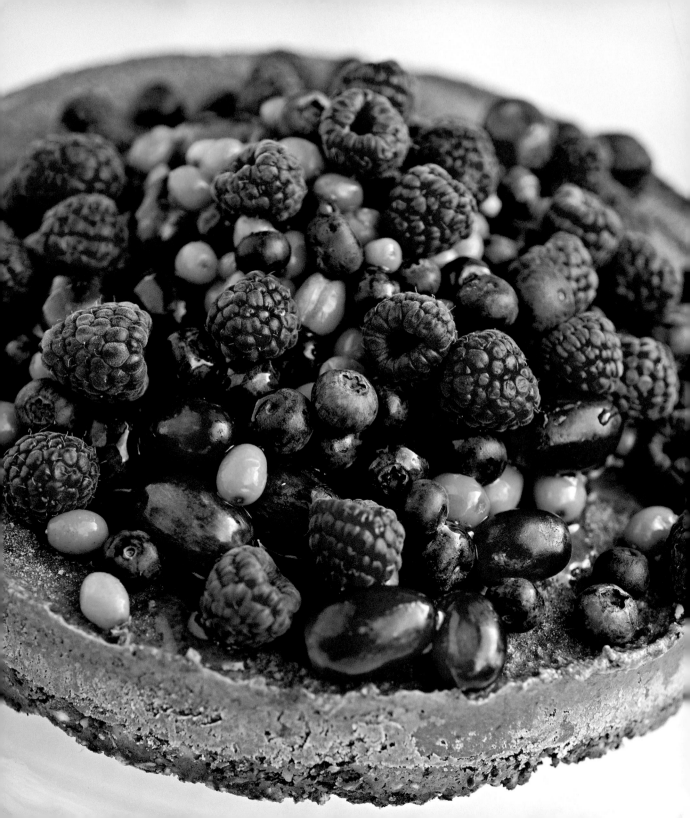

Yoga Cake

Man, you will love this cake! I make it often, in all possible variations. It contains good fats and is not too sweet, but it will fill you up nicely. Buckthorn is perfect, with its acid cutting through the sweet cake, or you can use orange slices. Don't let it sit out too long at room temperature or it will melt.

About 12 servings

2 cups (500 ml) almonds, soaked for 4 hours

2 cups (500 ml) dried dates, soaked for 4 hours

2 tbsp cocoa

1 tsp vanilla seeds or 1 tsp ground vanilla bean

2 cups (500 ml) cashews, soaked for 4 hours

2 bananas

2 tsp ground cardamom

1/2 cup (100 ml) agave nectar

4 tbsp coconut oil

about 1/4 cup (50 ml) juice of 1 lemon

2 cups (500 ml) raspberries (about 1 lb
    [450 g] frozen)

1 tsp sea salt

fresh fruits and berries for garnish, preferably
    sea buckthorn or orange slices

DIRECTIONS:

1. Cover the bottom of a springform pan with plastic wrap.

2. Mix almonds, pitted dates, cocoa, and vanilla bean into a crumbly dough. Flatten into the bottom of the pan.

3. Mix cashew nuts, banana, cardamom, agave nectar, coconut oil, lemon juice, raspberries, and salt into a smooth paste. It may take some time to get the right consistency.

4. Pour the pulp on top of the dough. Cover with plastic wrap and set the mixture in the freezer for at least 4 hours. You can also bake the cake the day before serving, put it in the freezer, and let it soften in the refrigerator for 1–2 hours before serving.

5. Garnish with (grapes, blueberries, raspberries, or sea buckthorn, available frozen, or orange slices) to serve.

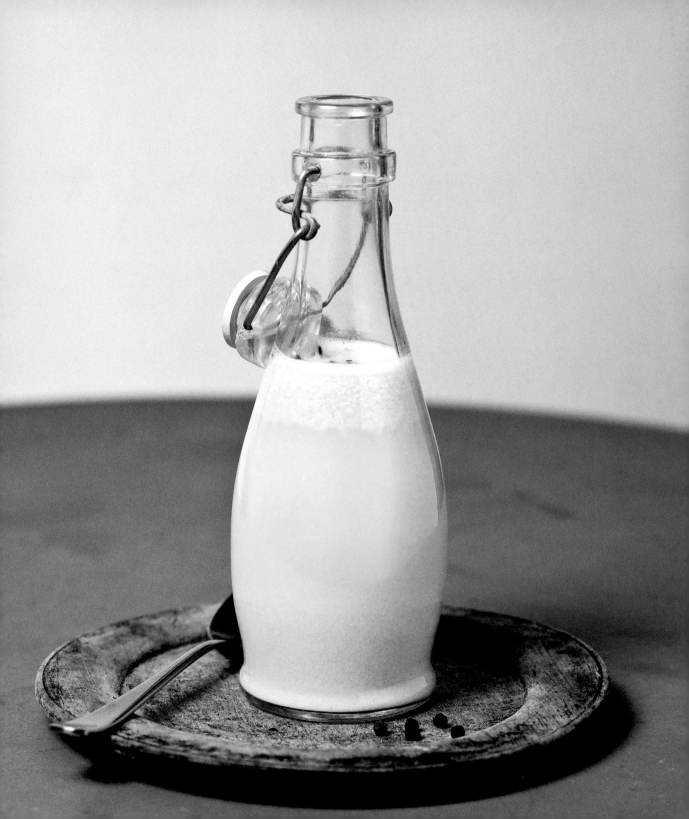

Ginger Elixir

Pepper, lemon, and ginger. Hot, strengthening, and great for getting your digestive system going. Stir about a tbsp into a glass of water and drink before you eat lunch and dinner. You can really feel how it purifies while boosting your immune system!

A hefty piece of ginger (fist-sized)

4 lemons

2 limes

3 tbsp honey

1 scant cup (200 ml) water

10 black peppercorns

DIRECTIONS:

1. Cut the ginger into 1/2 inch (1 cm)-sized pieces and juice it in a juice extractor to make about 1/2 cup (100 ml) juice. Or you can grate the ginger and squeeze out the juice.

2. Squeeze the lemon and lime. Mix juices and whisk in the honey, water, and black pepper.

3. Store in a pitcher in the fridge.

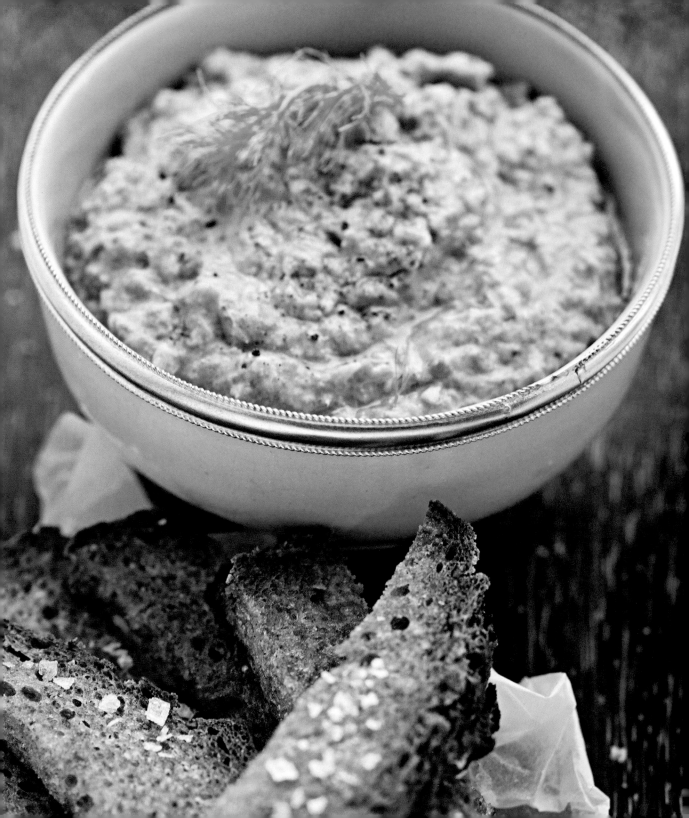

Fennel Dip

This is a perfect dip to keep in the fridge, to use as a topping on your late-night sandwich after yoga, or to flavor any dish at all. You can also do as we do here and serve with crusty sourdough breadsticks as an appetizer or snack.

1 fennel

olive oil

1 tsp fennel seeds

1 scant cup (200 ml) cooked mung beans, green lentils, or any kind of beans

1 tbsp tahini

1 clove garlic

2 tbsp tamari

1 tbsp apple cider vinegar

1/2–1 tsp Tabasco (preferably green jalapeño Tabasco sauce)

sea salt flakes

black pepper

2 tbsp water, if needed

DIRECTIONS:

1. Preheat the oven to 400°F (200°C). Coarsely chop the fennel. Place the pieces on a plate and add 1–2 tbsp of olive oil. Roast until golden, about 20 minutes.

2. Toast the fennel seeds in a dry, hot pan then grind them with a mortar and pestle.

3. Mix the fennel in a food processor together with mung beans, tahini, chopped garlic, fennel seeds, tamari, apple cider vinegar, and Tabasco. Season with salt and pepper and possibly add some water for a looser consistency.

SOURDOUGH BREADSTICKS

Cut long breadsticks out of sourdough bread. Heat up coconut oil or olive oil in a pan and toast the bread. Sprinkle with salt flakes.

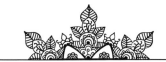

Tip! Always have a tasty dip in the fridge! It can be put on sandwiches, used to dip oven-roasted vegetables, or smeared on crackers. It makes you less tempted to eat something unhealthy.

51

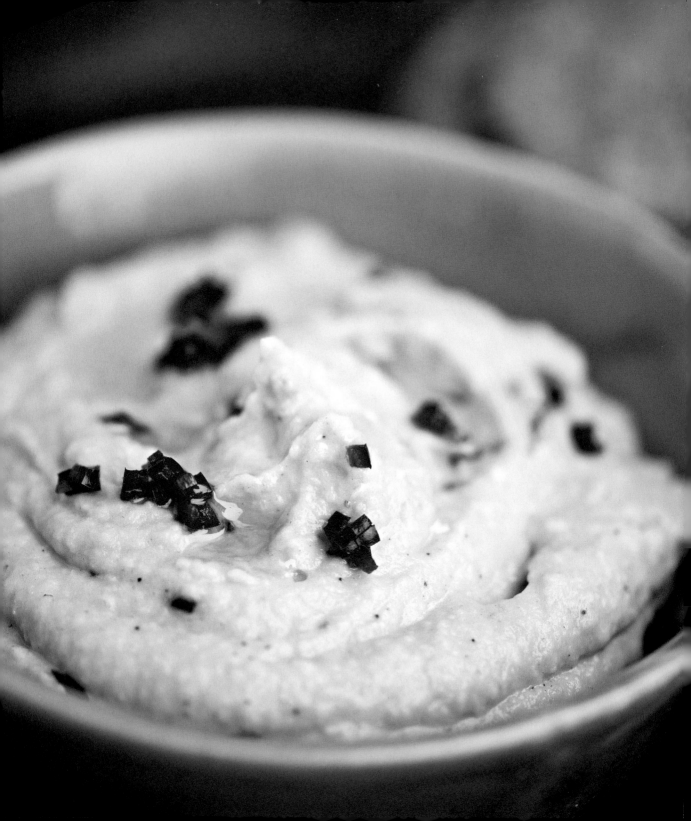

Jerusalem Artichoke Hummus

This is a very useful, fluffy, and smooth dip that can be served with crackers, as a filling for a sandwich, or on a salad. Good also with fish!

about 5 oz (150 g) Jerusalem artichokes (approximately 2 pieces)
1–1 1/2 cup (200–300 ml) cooked large white beans (about 1 14–15 oz can)
juice and zest of 1/2 lemon
1 tsp tahini
2 tbsp olive oil
1 clove garlic
1/2 chili pepper
sea salt and black pepper

DIRECTIONS:
1. Peel artichokes down to the hearts under running water. Cut the artichoke hearts into pieces and boil them until soft (about 15 minutes). Allow to cool.
2. Mix artichoke hearts with beans, lemon, tahini, olive oil, garlic, and chopped chili pepper. Season with sea salt and black pepper.

Serve with crackers or vegetables.

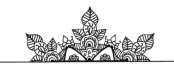

Tip! Fried Jerusalem artichokes are also good! Clean the artichoke hearts under running water. Cut into thin slices and fry in coconut oil. Sprinkle with salt if you like and serve as a snack.

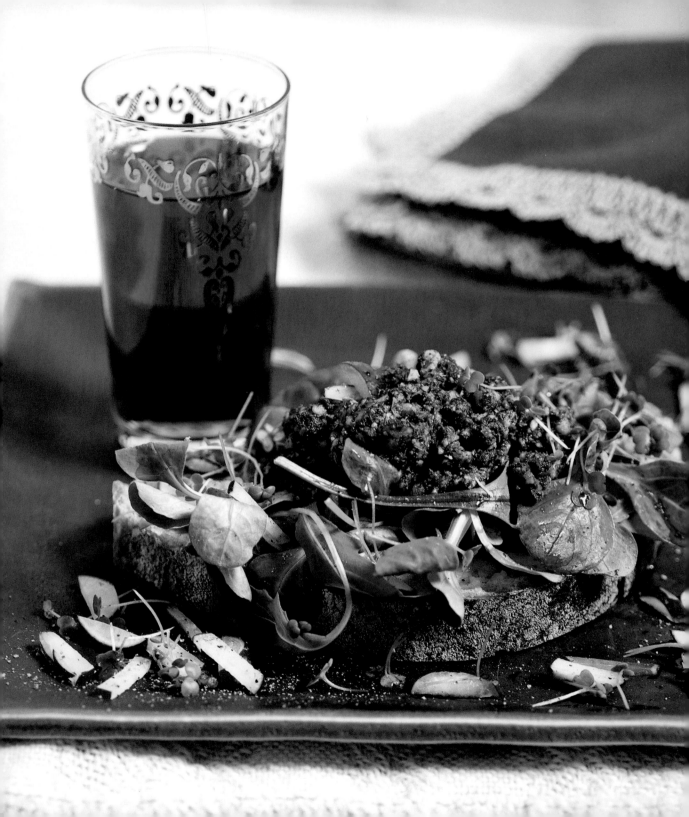

Pistachio Pesto

Creamy, tasty, and crunchy! Serve as a spread, or put a dollop in a soup or stew. You can also mix it with beans, or serve with steamed fish, freshly cooked pasta, or quinoa.

1 garlic clove
2 bunches basil
3/4 cup (150 ml) shelled pistachios
1/2 cup (100 ml) olive oil
1/2 tsp sea salt
a few turns with the pepper mill

DIRECTIONS:

1. Peel and mince the garlic. Combine the remainder of the ingredients into a coarsely chopped mixture and add the garlic.
2. If you use the pesto as a sandwich spread, you could serve it on a nice slice of sourdough bread with chopped radish and sprouts.

Seed Topping

This topping will increase the nutrient density of your lunch salad in a snap, giving you lots of wonderfully toasted crunch.

(The seed sprinkle is not pictured.)

1 scant cup (200 ml) pumpkin seeds
1/2 cup (100 ml) sesame seeds
3 tbsp tamari
1 tsp coriander seeds, dried and ground
1 tsp apple cider vinegar

DIRECTIONS:

1. Preheat the oven to 350°F (175°C).
2. Mix all ingredients in a bowl and spread on a baking sheet lined with parchment paper.
3. Roast for 35 minutes.
4. Let cool slightly before serving. Store the seeds in a jar with a lid.

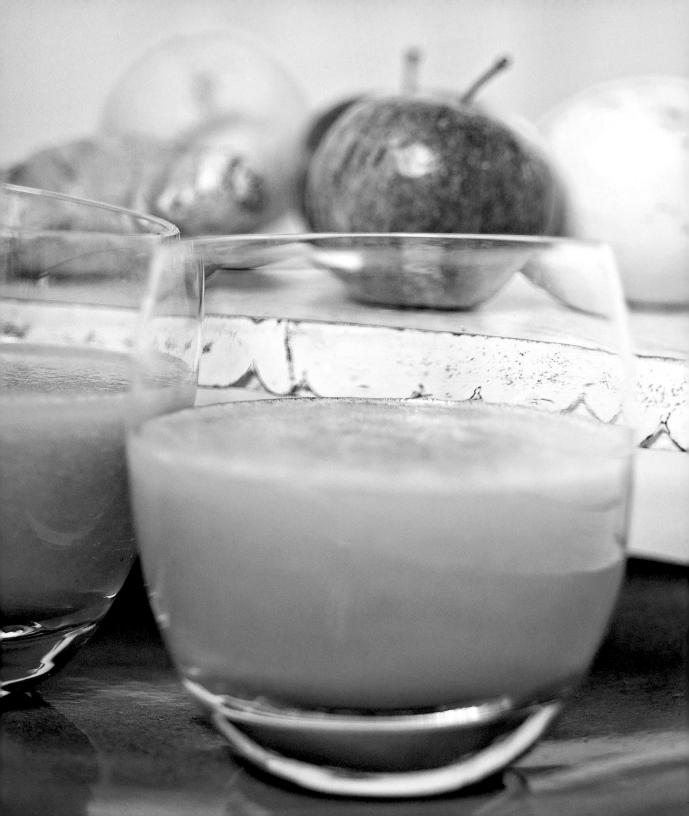

Chlorophyll Juice

A real kick-start whenever you need it! Incredibly tasty and very healthy, with a fresh flavor and a little heat from the ginger.

1 large glass
3 apples
1 thumb-sized piece of ginger
2 stalks celery
1 bunch parsley
juice of 1 lemon

DIRECTIONS:

1. Juice the apples and ginger in a juice extractor.
2. In a blender, chop the celery into pieces with parsley. Add the apple and ginger juice and season to taste with lemon juice.

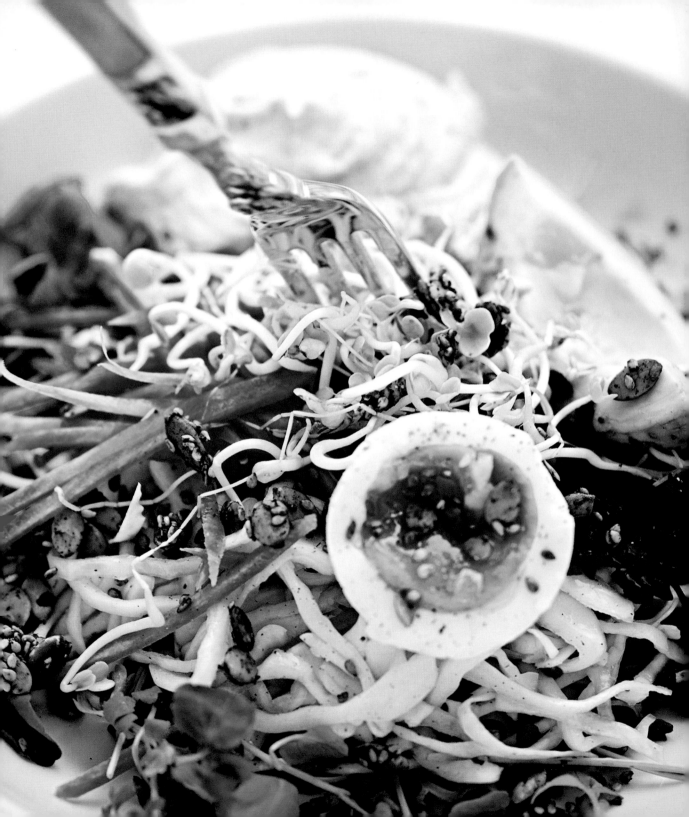

Yoga Salad

This salad is a perfect lunch or dinner after a yoga class. It is fresh, crunchy, and very filling and satisfying, depending on what you serve with it. If you are not able to get the fermented red cabbage, you can use other fermented cabbage, including kimchi.

1 serving
a generous wedge of cabbage
grated zest of 1/4 lemon
1 tsp apple cider vinegar
2 tbsp olive oil
sea salt and black pepper
1/2 carrot
3 tbsp lacto-fermented red cabbage
1/4 cup (50 ml) toasted nuts and seeds
1 handful of sprouts
1/2 avocado

Serving suggestions: cheese, boiled eggs, leafy greens, mixed beans, and bread.

DIRECTIONS:

1. Shred the cabbage. Mix cabbage, lemon zest, apple cider vinegar, and olive oil in a bowl. Add about 1 pinch of salt and 1 pinch of pepper and rub into the cabbage.

2. Peel and shred the carrot. Add the carrot, fermented red cabbage, nuts and seeds, sprouts, and avocado in pieces in a wide bowl with the cabbage.

3. Serve with a piece of cheese, eggs, leafy greens, mixed beans, or bread, depending on how hungry you are.

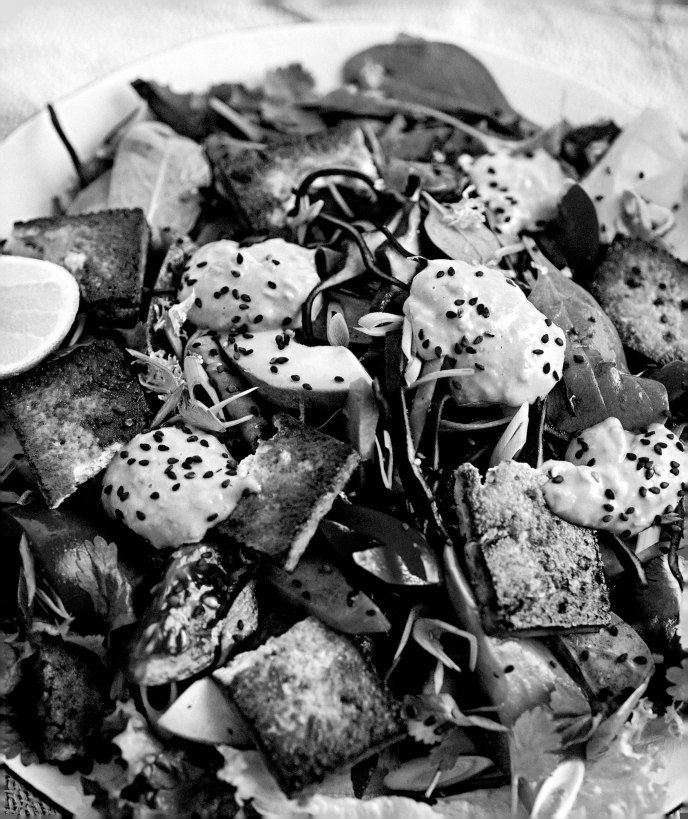

Gado-Gado—Indonesian Salad with Peanut Sauce

This is a classic Indonesian dish that I was inspired by when I worked at a retreat in Bali—Kumara Sakti. Balinese food is wonderful, with lots of peanuts, tropical fruits, lime, cilantro, tofu, and tempeh . . . yummy!

4 servings

7 oz (200 g) firm tofu

2 tbsp + 1–2 tbsp tamari

1 tbsp + 1 tbsp grated ginger

1 tsp Tabasco

1/2 cup (100 ml) peanut butter or roasted peanuts

1/4 leek

1/2 chili pepper

juice and grated zest of 3 limes

salt and pepper

1/2 red cabbage

1 bell pepper

3 spring onions

2 tomatoes

2 avocados

1 3/4 oz (50 g) spinach

1/2–1 papaya or mango

1 bunch cilantro

coconut oil or olive oil for frying

optional: sesame seeds for garnish

DIRECTIONS:

1. Cut the tofu into slices and marinate in 2 tbsp soy sauce, 1 tbsp grated ginger, and Tabasco.

2. Mix peanuts, 1 tbsp grated ginger, coarsely sliced leeks, chopped chili pepper, 1–2 tbsp soy sauce, and the peel and juice from 2 limes. Dilute with a little water if needed and add salt and pepper. Set the sauce aside.

3. Shred cabbage and peppers. Slice the spring onions thinly. Cut the tomatoes into chunks and the avocado into wedges. Divide with spinach on a large platter or four individual serving dishes.

4. Cut papaya into cubes and mix with the juice and grated zest of the remaining lime. Spread this over the salad and top with coarsely chopped cilantro.

5. Fry tofu in coconut oil over medium heat until golden.

Serve the salad with tofu and peanut sauce. If you like, sprinkle sesame seeds on top.

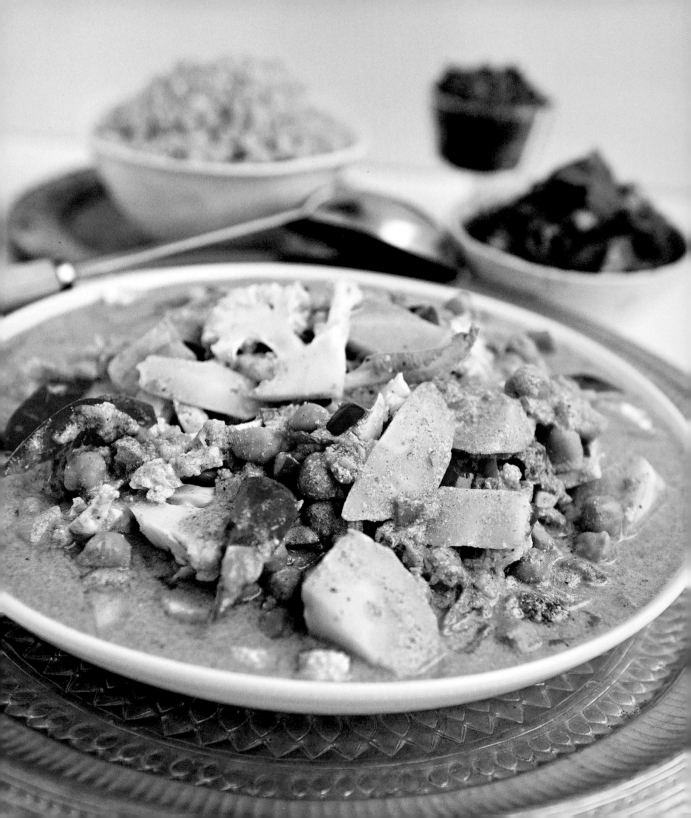

Indian Stew

A delicious stew with everything your body needs! No strange ingredients, but very tasty.

4 servings

6 cloves garlic

1 piece ginger, thumb-sized

1 onion

2 chili peppers

2 parsnips

4 tomatoes

olive oil and butter for frying

3 tbsp Indian spice mixture (see recipe in the next section), or 2 tbsp garam masala

2 cups (500 ml) whole-milk yogurt

2 tbsp vegetable bouillon powder

1 scant cup (200 ml) water

1/2 cauliflower head

1 red bell pepper

1 can of any beans, 1 1/2–1 3/4 cups (300–400 ml) cooked

1 lime

sea salt

Serve with whole-grain basmati rice

DIRECTIONS:

1. Peel the garlic, ginger, and onion, and chop finely with the chili pepper.

2. Peel the parsnips and cut into pieces. Cut the tomatoes coarsely.

3. Heat 2 tbsp butter and 2 tbsp olive oil in a pan with high edges. Add the garlic, ginger, onion, and chili pepper, and stir while cooking.

4. Add the parsnips and spices or garam masala and stir. Add the tomatoes, yogurt, bouillon powder, and water and let sit for a minute. Next bring to a boil and simmer for 10 minutes.

5. Rinse and clean the cauliflower (peel the stem as well and use it). Seed the peppers and cut into small pieces. Rinse the beans.

6. Add vegetables and beans to the pot. Bring to a boil and simmer for another 5 minutes.

7. Grate the zest and squeeze the juice from the lime. Season with salt and serve with fruit chutney (page 68) and whole-grain basmati rice.

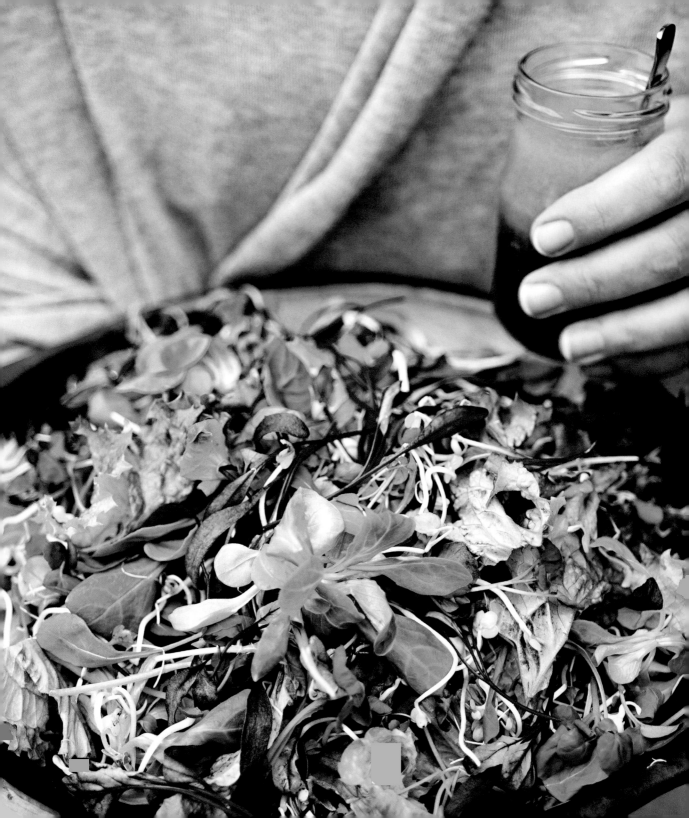

Happiness Dressing

A simple green salad can be lifted to unprecedented heights with this dressing on top. It can also flavor cabbage and leafy greens, and it has an immune-boosting effect.

1 clove garlic

1/2 cup (100 ml) lemon juice
(about 2 lemons)

1 tbsp finely grated ginger

3 tbsp tamari

1/2 tbsp agave nectar (or maple syrup)

1/2 cup (100 ml) olive oil

DIRECTIONS:

1. Grate the garlic and mix with the rest of the ingredients in a glass jar with lid.
2. Shake and serve. The dressing will keep for 2 weeks in the fridge.

Indian Spice Mix

All the spices in this blend have invigorating and stimulating properties, but turmeric has an extra superpower—it is a protective antioxidant and has anti-inflammatory properties.

1 tbsp ground coriander

1 tsp ground ginger

1 tbsp ground cumin

1 tbsp mustard seeds

1 tsp turmeric

1 tsp cinnamon

1/4 tsp cayenne pepper

DIRECTIONS:

1. Grind the dry spices using a mortar and pestle and store what is not needed right away in a jar with a lid. The mixture is enough for a couple of Indian dishes.

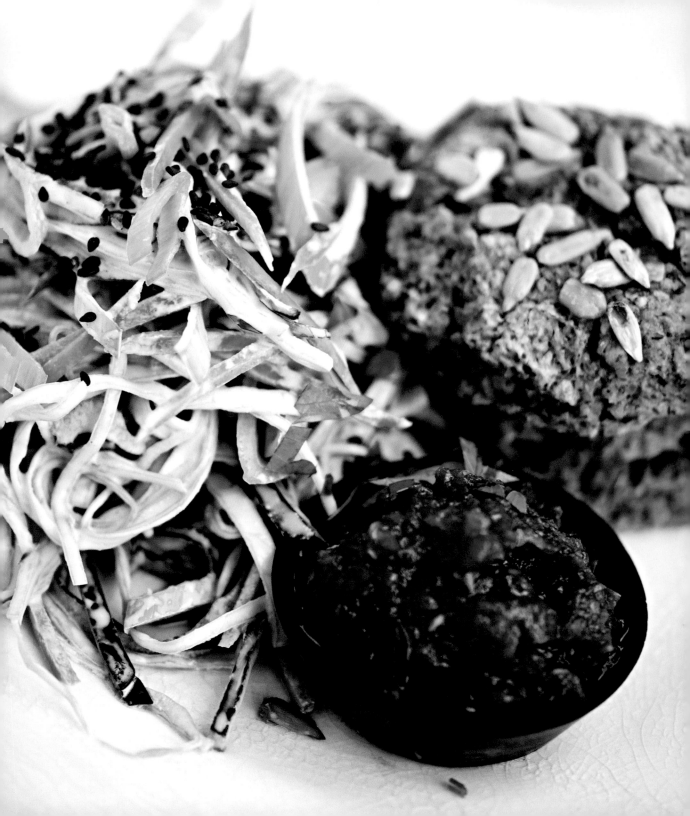

Green Falafel

Chickpeas are rich in protein and have a lovely texture when you mash them and make patties of the mixture.

About 14 pieces

1 red onion

2 shallots

1 bunch cilantro

1 bunch parsley

1/2 bunch dill

1 tsp sambal oelek

sea salt

2 cloves garlic

1 scant cup (200 ml) green peas

1 3/4 cups (400 ml) chickpeas, cooked

1 tsp baking powder

coconut oil for brushing

seeds, such as pumpkin seeds, sesame seeds, or sunflower seeds

DIRECTIONS:

1. Preheat the oven to 400°F (200°C). Peel and chop the onion and shallots. Mix together with herbs, sambal oelek, and 1/2 tsp salt in a food processor.

2. Add the grated garlic, green peas, and chickpeas, and blend to a coarse but smooth mixture. Place the mixture in a bowl and stir in baking powder.

3. Shape into balls or patties. The batter will be quite loose. Place on a cookie sheet lined with parchment paper. Brush with melted coconut oil and sprinkle with seeds. Bake in the middle of the oven for 30–40 minutes.

4. Serve with cabbage salad and tomato sauce (see the next section) or maybe with a lacto-fermented vegetable and leafy greens.

Fresh Tomato Sauce

A classic sauce that is good for everything from roasted vegetables to the falafel patties on page 67.

4 tomatoes

1/2 yellow onion or 4 inches (10 cm) leek

6 sun-dried tomatoes, soaked

1 bunch basil or cilantro

10 drops Tabasco or
   1/2 tsp sambal oelek

1 tbsp tamari

1 tsp agave nectar or honey

DIRECTIONS:

1. Blanch and peel tomatoes. Peel and chop the onion roughly.
2. Place all ingredients in a blender and blend to a smooth sauce. Season to taste and serve.

Fruit Chutney

A great-tasting chutney that does not require any cooking and that is super-yummy with all kinds of stews and casseroles.

10 dried apricots, preferably soaked
   for 4 hours

6 dried figs, preferably soaked for 4 hours

1/2 yellow onion

1/2 bunch cilantro

1/2 tsp sea salt

3 tbsp olive oil

2 tbsp apple cider vinegar

DIRECTIONS:

1. Finely chop the apricots and figs and mix together in a bowl.
2. Peel and finely chop the onion. Chop the cilantro. Mix with the dried fruit and add salt, olive oil, and apple cider vinegar. Set in a cool place to serve.

Coleslaw

Eat more cabbage! You can use any kind you want: kale, broccoli, cauliflower . . . Cabbage contains vitamin C, strengthens the immune system, and is purifying.

4 servings

1/2 small head of cabbage, or equivalent
   amount of other cabbage

sea salt

1 large carrot

1/2 cup (100 ml) pine nuts or cashews

1 tbsp red wine vinegar

3/4 cup cold-pressed sesame oil or olive oil

juice and finely shredded zest of 1/2 lemon

1 tsp Dijon mustard

roasted seeds as a garnish, such as sesame

DIRECTIONS:

1. Shred the cabbage very thin. Rinse it and let it drain. Place in a bowl and rub in 1/2 tsp salt. Let sit for 10 minutes.
2. Peel and cut carrots into thin strips. Add them to the bowl.
3. Mix the nuts with vinegar, oil, lemon juice, zest, and mustard. Add salt.
4. Mix the dressing with cabbage and carrot. Garnish with seeds.

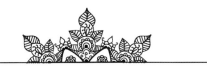

Tip! What are enzymes?
Enzymes are small protein parts. The enzyme production of the body begins when we eat. Food enzymes that we can provide for the body are found in raw fruits, raw vegetables, and sprouts.

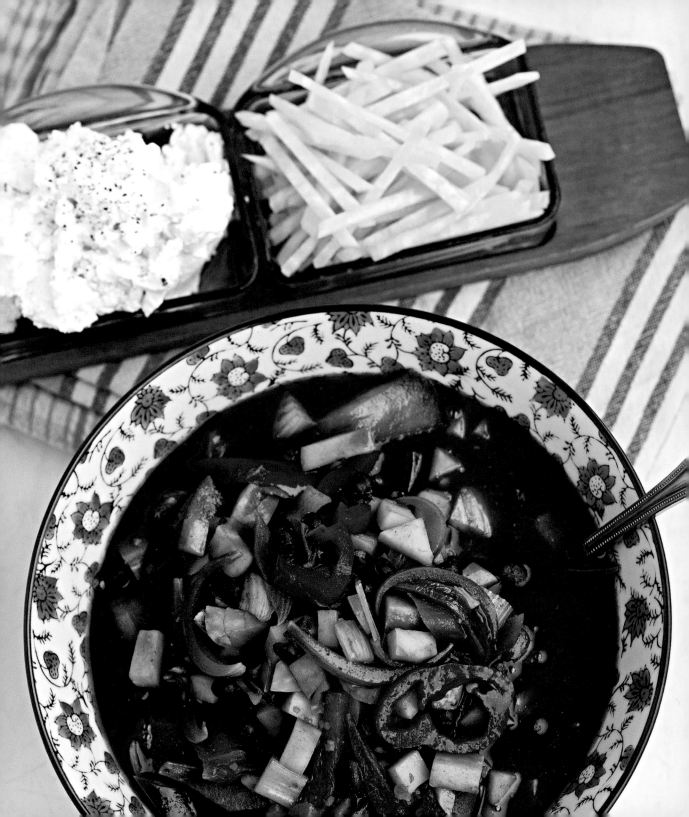

Smoky Vegetable Stew with Black Beans

This is a good dinner that is perfect for putting in the lunch box the next day. The smoky chipotle chili is perfect for adding variety to the vegetarian food. You can use chipotle Tabasco, or crushed or whole chipotle that you mince.

4 servings

1 red onion

3 cloves garlic

1/2 celeriac, about 10 1/2 oz (300 g)

1 fennel

1/2 eggplant

1 bell pepper

2 tbsp coconut oil or olive oil

1 tsp paprika

1 tsp ground cumin

2 tbsp tomato paste

1 scant cup (200 ml) red wine

2 cups (500 ml) water

2 tbsp vegetable bouillon powder

2 tsp chipotle Tabasco or 1 tsp ground dried chipotle chili peppers

1 1/2 cup (300 ml) cooked black beans (about 1 14–15 oz can)

juice of 1/2 lemon

1 tsp honey

2 tbsp tamari

sea salt and black pepper

DIRECTIONS:

1. Peel the onion, garlic, and celeriac. Cut the onion. Finely chop the garlic. Cut the celeriac into pieces. Cut the fennel, eggplant, and bell pepper into small pieces.

2. Heat oil in a large pot, preferably cast iron. Fry onion, garlic, and celeriac for a few minutes and then add the remaining vegetables and stir. Let fry for 5–8 minutes.

3. Add bell pepper, coriander, and tomato paste, and stir. Add the red wine, water, bouillon powder, and chipotle pepper. Put on the lid and bring to a boil. Simmer for about 10 minutes.

4. Add the beans, lemon juice, honey, and tamari. Season with salt and pepper. Set the pot to the lowest heat for a few minutes until the flavors are combined.

5. Serve the stew with finely shredded raw yellow beet and a sauce made with sheep's cheese, sour cream, black pepper, olive oil, and, if you like, some whole-grain rice.

71

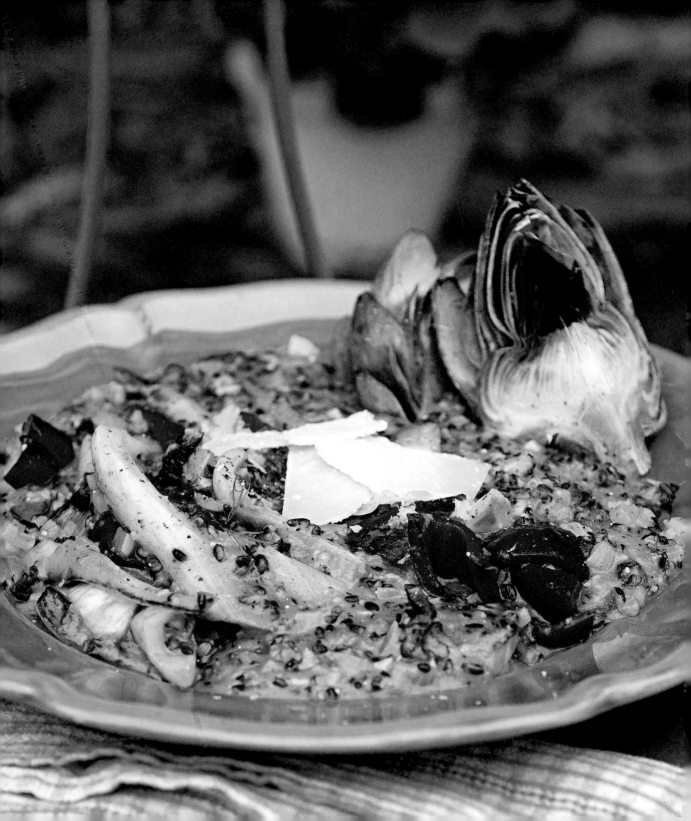

Yoga Risotto

A wonderfully creamy and flavorful risotto that is quick to make if you have precooked rice in the fridge—cook a big batch of rice for this dish the day before!

4 servings

1 onion

4 cloves garlic

2 stalks celery

3 tbsp olive oil

10 sun-dried tomatoes

about 2 1/2 cups (600 ml) cooked brown rice (about 1 1/2 cup [300 ml] uncooked)

1 scant cup (200 ml) white wine or cooking wine

1 scant cup (200 ml) water

2–3 tbsp vegetable bouillon powder

juice and zest of 1/2 lemon

1 tbsp butter

1/2 cup (100 ml) grated Parmesan

black pepper

1 fennel

1 bell pepper

1 tbsp olive oil

salt

DIRECTIONS:

1. Peel and finely chop the onion and garlic. Finely chop the celery. Heat olive oil in a heavy-bottomed saucepan and fry onion, garlic, and celery over medium heat until the onion has softened.

2. Chop the sun-dried tomatoes. Add the cooked brown rice, sun-dried tomatoes, wine, water, and bouillon powder. Bring to a boil and simmer for 5–8 minutes until the risotto has thickened.

3. Add the lemon, butter, Parmesan, and black pepper. Leave on low heat.

4. Cut the fennel into thin slices and the bell pepper into thick strips. Fry in olive oil in a frying pan. Season with salt and pepper. Stir into the risotto.

5. Serve the risotto on a large plate, and top it with artichoke and more Parmesan.

BOILED ARTICHOKE

Boil an artichoke heart for about 30 minutes. Cut it into wedges and mix it with a little olive oil, balsamic vinegar, salt, and pepper. Or shred four grilled artichoke hearts from a can and mix around in the marinade.

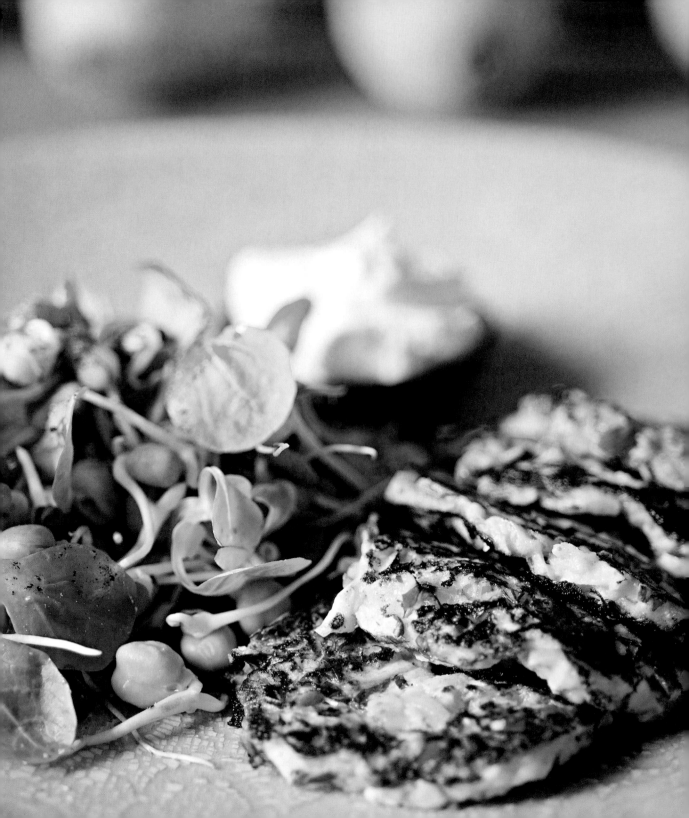

Zucchini Fritters

These are super good! And they are filled with hearty vegetables that will fill you up.

Approximately 25 pieces
2 zucchinis
sea salt
2 yellow onions
5 garlic cloves
3 tbsp olive oil
3 eggs
3 tbsp spelt flour
7 oz (200 g) feta cheese or 31/2 oz
    (100 g) Parmesan
1 bunch Italian parsley
1/2 bunch mint
1 bunch dill
1/2 tsp Tabasco
coconut oil or butter and olive oil for frying

DIRECTIONS:

1. Grate the zucchini coarsely. Place in a colander with 1 tsp sea salt. Set aside and let the liquid drain.
2. Peel and finely chop the onion and garlic. Heat the olive oil and fry the onion and garlic gently until soft.
3. Beat the eggs lightly with spelt flour and crumble the cheese into the mixture. Chop the herbs finely and mix.
4. Add the onion, hot sauce, 1 tsp sea salt, and 2 pinches of pepper.
5. Squeeze out as much liquid as you can from the zucchini. Fold the zucchini into the egg batter. Let batter rest for 5 minutes.
6. Heat the coconut oil in a frying pan or a crepe pan. Fry small pancakes on medium heat. Serve with a big salad and a yogurt dipping sauce.

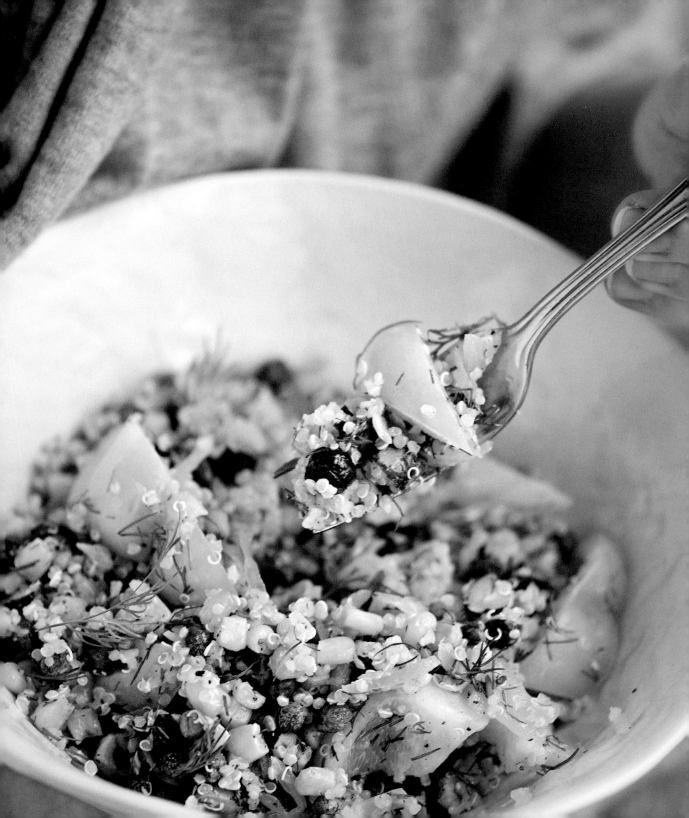

Healthy Dish

A bowl of nutrition! Quinoa is easily digested and rich in protein—you will be completely satisfied! It's also good to bring in a lunch box for work or on a train ride—it stays fresh for a long time. The hazelnuts may be replaced with almonds.

1–2 servings

1/2 cup (100 ml) hazelnuts

1 1/2 cup (300 ml) raw corn kernels

1 tbsp coconut oil

1 tsp dried sage

sea salt

1 bell pepper

1 1/2 cup (300 ml) cooked grains, such
   as quinoa

1/2 cup (100 ml) sauerkraut or lacto-fermented
   red cabbage for a sweeter flavor

1/4 cup (50 ml) finely chopped dill

juice and grated zest of 1/2 lemon

2 tbsp olive oil

2 tsp vegetable bouillon powder

3 tbsp capers

black pepper

DIRECTIONS:

1. Preheat the oven to 350°F (175°C). Coarsely chop the hazelnuts. Spread corn, hazelnuts, coconut oil, sage, and a pinch of sea salt in an oven-proof pan. Roast in the oven for 15 minutes. Allow to cool.

2. Cut pepper into small pieces. Mix the grains with pepper, sauerkraut, dill, lemon, olive oil, bouillon powder, and capers. Season with sea salt and black pepper.

3. Fold the nut mixture into the salad.

Tip! Fast food for yogis: Cooked quinoa that you mix with roasted vegetables and serve with a yummy sauce on top!

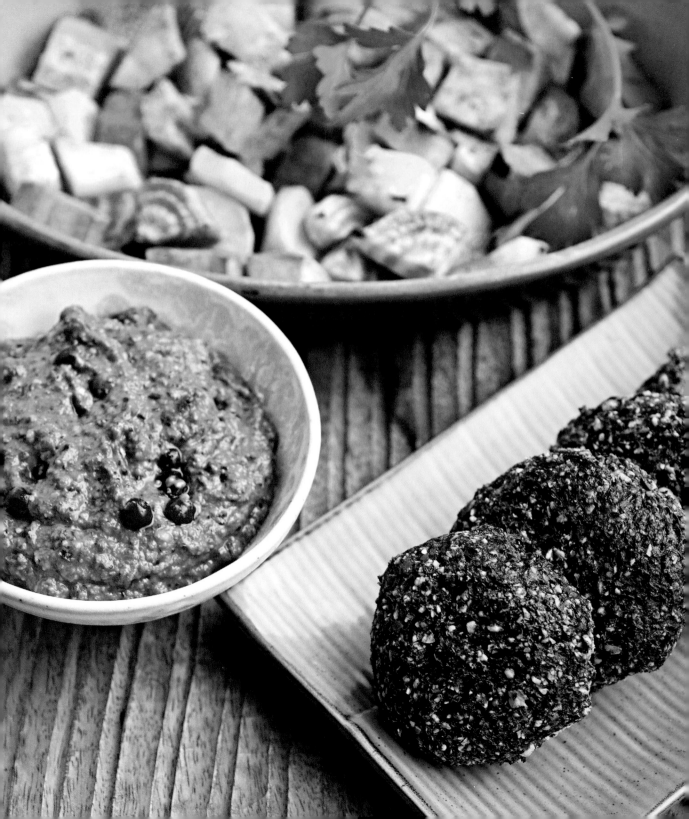

Mushroom Burger

Mushrooms are a good option for getting a bit of variation when you eat vegetarian food. You can use everything from freshly picked chanterelles to organically grown white button mushrooms, depending on the season.

8 medium-sized burgers
olive oil
2 large portobello mushrooms, chopped
2 cups (500 ml) parboiled mushrooms, any kind, cleaned and finely chopped
1/2 sweet potato, peeled and finely grated
1 large onion, peeled and chopped
4 cloves garlic, peeled and chopped
1 scant cup (200 ml) cashews
1/2 cup (100 ml) pumpkin seeds
3 tbsp finely chopped chives
3 tbsp light miso paste or tamari
2 tsp lemon juice
black pepper
1 scant cup grain (200 ml) such as buckwheat, quinoa, amaranth, or millet

DIRECTIONS:
1. Heat about 1 tbsp olive oil in a frying pan and fry the mushrooms. Add the onion and garlic and cook, stirring for about 5 minutes.
2. Add sweet potato and cook an additional 5 minutes. Allow to cool.
3. Mix nuts and pumpkin seeds. Add the mushroom mixture, chives, miso paste, lemon juice, 2 pinches of black pepper, and grains. Pulse mixture to a coarse consistency. Let stand for several hours in the fridge.
4. Preheat the oven to 400°F (200°C). Spoon out the batter onto a baking sheet with parchment paper. Drizzle with olive oil and roast in the oven for about 30 minutes.
5. Serve with, for example, oven-roasted root vegetables and lingonberry chutney.

LINGONBERRY CHUTNEY
[Note: Raw lingonberries can be difficult to obtain outside of Sweden; however, they are similar in taste and texture to cranberries.]
A tasty and hot condiment for everything that goes well with lingonberries: steaks, burgers, fritters.

1/2 red onion, peeled and coarsely chopped
1/2 chili pepper, chopped
1/2 cup (100 ml) cashews
1/2 cup (100 ml) lingonberries
1 tsp honey
1 tbsp apple cider vinegar
salt

DIRECTIONS:
1. Mix the ingredients. Season with salt and stir in some whole lingonberries at the end.

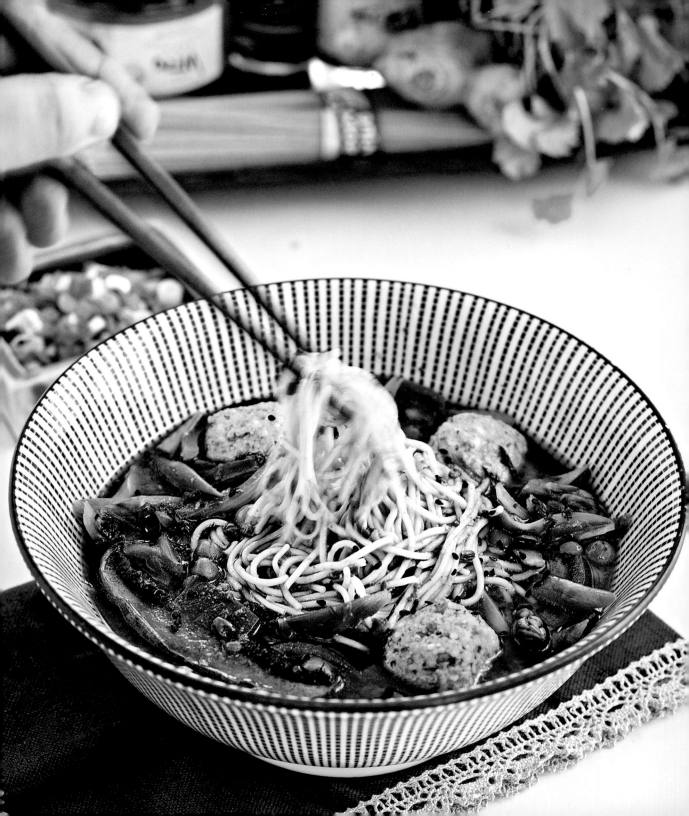

Japanese Clear Soup with Ginger and Soba Noodles

Warm, simple, and absolutely delicious after a strenuous yoga class! In fact, it's actually like fast food, if you make the quenelles or serve with large white beans. Noodles come in all varieties—pick your own favorite. Mine are brown rice, buckwheat, and sweet potato noodles.

4 servings

1 package of soba noodles, 7 oz (200 g),
   or other noodles

1 red onion

1 piece ginger

1 tbsp coconut oil

3 1/2 cups (800 ml) water

2 tbsp rice wine vinegar (mirin)

10 shiitake mushrooms

8 asparagus spears or 1 zucchini

1 scant cup (200 ml) green peas

4 tbsp miso paste, medium brown,
   or barley miso

1 tsp Tabasco, preferably green

16 spinach quenelles (see recipe on next page)
   or a 14–15 oz (400 g) can large white beans

Topping: 2 scallions, seeds, and coriander.

DIRECTIONS:

1. Cook the noodles according to the directions on the package. They should be al dente.

2. Peel and slice the onion. Peel and mince the ginger. Heat the coconut oil in a saucepan and fry the ginger and onion until soft. Add water and rice vinegar and boil. Simmer for 5 minutes.

3. Shred the shiitakes and cut the asparagus into pieces. Add this and the peas and simmer for another 5 minutes.

4. Put aside about 1/2 cup (100 ml) broth in a bowl and mix with the miso paste till it dissolves. Add and mix well. Season with Tabasco.

5. Heat quenelles (see next page) or beans (liquid drained) in the soup with finely shredded scallions, seeds, and coriander.

Spinach Quenelles

Beautiful little green balls that can be served in soup or maybe in a tomato sauce with noodles or brown rice. The parsnip can be replaced with Jerusalem artichokes, carrots, or sweet potatoes.

About 16 pieces
1 parsnip
1 3/4 oz (50 g) spinach
1 scant cup (200 ml) cashews or almonds
1 egg
finely grated zest of 1/2 lemon
1/2 cup (100 ml) millet flakes (or spelt or buckwheat flakes)
sea salt and black pepper
1 tbsp vegetable stock powder

DIRECTIONS:

1. Peel and cut the parsnip into small cubes. Boil until soft, about 5 minutes.

2. Mix spinach, nuts, eggs, lemon zest, flakes, parsnip, 1/2 tsp salt, and 2 pinches pepper quickly into a batter. It should be a little coarse.

3. Use two spoons to shape the quenelles. Boil 2 cups (500 ml) water and add the vegetable bouillon powder. Drop in a few quenelles at a time and simmer for about 5 minutes.

4. Serve in soup, as on page 81.

Lentil Soup

A soup with lots of vegetables and a flavor that will be even better with toppings such as feta or chèvre, grated Parmesan cheese, sprouts, eggs, sourdough croutons, nuts, seeds, leafy greens, olives, and capers.

4 servings

2 garlic cloves

1 piece ginger

1 onion

1 sweet potato or carrot

1 yellow bell pepper

1 fennel

1 tomato

2 tbsp of coconut oil

3 1/2 cups (800 ml) water

1 scant cup (200 ml) red lentils

1 tsp dried thyme

1 tsp dried rosemary

1 tsp dried sage

1 tbsp vegetable stock powder

2 tbsp apple cider vinegar

1 tsp sambal oelek

sea salt flakes and pepper

optional toppings

DIRECTIONS:

1. Peel and chop the garlic and ginger. Peel and cut onions and sweet potatoes into rough chunks. Chop the pepper and fennel coarsely. Cut the tomato into pieces.

2. Heat the coconut oil in a pan. Fry onions, garlic, and ginger. Lower to medium heat and add the remaining vegetables. Stir.

3. Add the water, lentils, herbs, bouillon powder, apple cider vinegar, and sambal oelek. Bring to a boil and simmer for 15 minutes. Season with salt and pepper. Serve with optional toppings and sourdough bread.

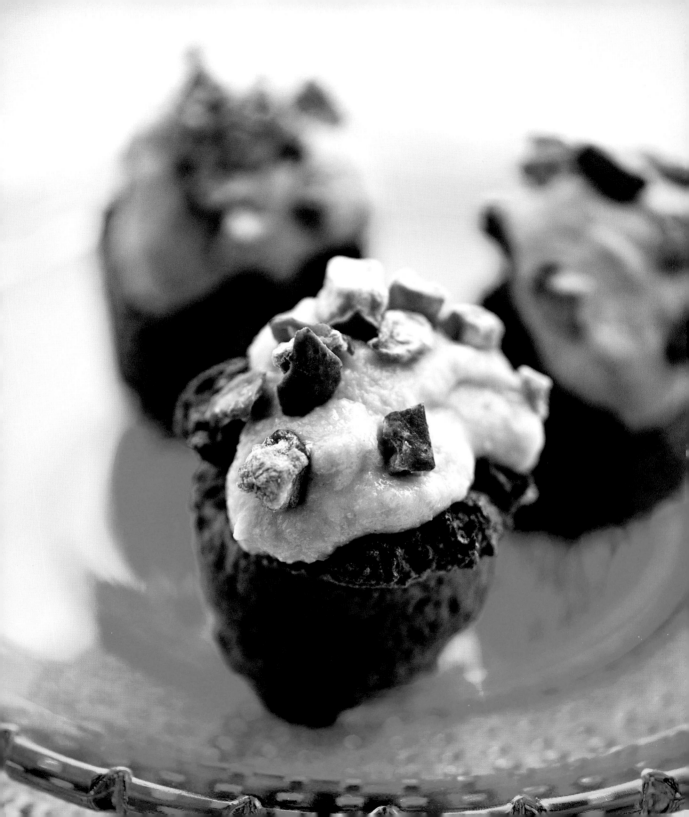

Nutty Banana Muffins

Sweet morning break muffins that will work just as well as a snack, since they contain hearty nuts.

About 15 small muffins

1 1/2 cup (300 ml) almonds

1 1/2 cup (300 ml) hazelnuts

1/2 cup (100 ml) coconut oil (or butter)

2 bananas

1/4 tsp ground allspice

3 tsp cinnamon

3 tsp ground cardamom

1/4 cup (50 ml) raisins, preferably
   soaked for 4 hours

1 pinch sea salt

DIRECTIONS:

1. Preheat the oven to 350°F (175°C). Mix almonds and hazelnuts in a food processor to a fine flour.

2. Add coconut oil, banana pieces, and other ingredients. Blend until smooth.

3. Spoon out the batter into mini muffin tins and bake for about 35 minutes.

4. Optional: Dollop with the apple topping and sprinkle with dried apple pieces, raisins, or goji berries.

APPLE TOPPING:

1 small apple

1/2 banana

1/2 cup (100 ml) cashews

DIRECTIONS:

1. Core the apple and slice it. Cut the banana into pieces. Mix the apple with the banana and cashew nuts into a smooth consistency.

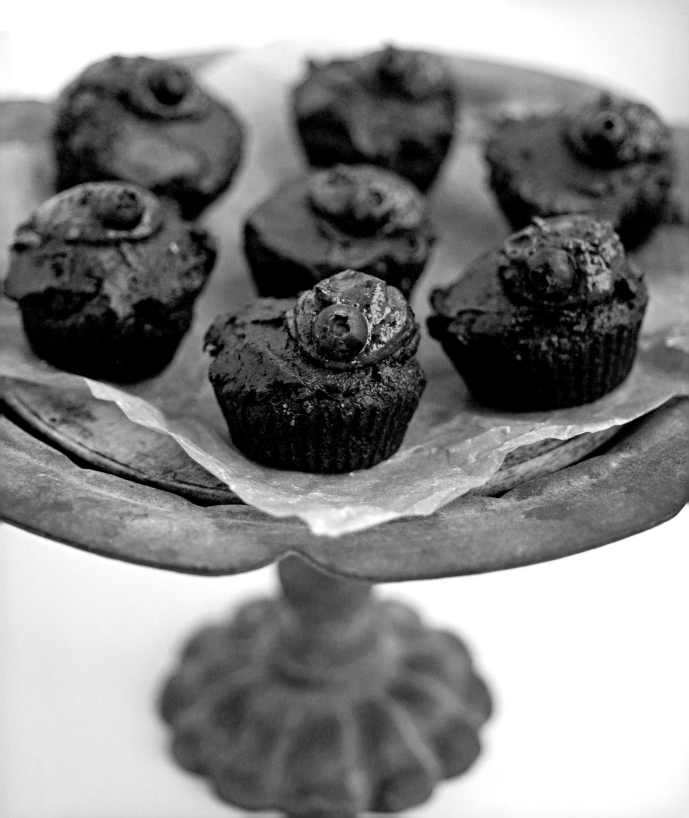

Chocolate Cake with Blueberry and Cashew Fluff

A delicious little treat! It contains no flour and is gluten-free. It is also eggless. This cake is so moist, and the dates provide natural sweetening. Fresh dates are a little larger and softer than dried ones and will give a fluffy consistency. Ten fresh dates correspond to approximately 15 dried and soaked. This is a nutrition bomb!

About 14 cakes

1 1/2 cup (300 ml) almonds

10 fresh dates

2 tsp ground cardamom

1/4 cup (50 ml) cocoa

3/8 cup (75 ml) coconut oil

1/2 vanilla bean

1 apple

1 1/2 cups (300 ml) blueberries

DIRECTIONS:

1. Preheat the oven to 350°F (175°C).
2. Mix the almonds into fine flour in the food processor. Add the pitted dates, cardamom, cocoa, and coconut oil.
3. Scrape the vanilla seeds from the vanilla pod and add to the mixture. Grate the apple coarsely and add that as well. Blend until smooth.
4. Add the blueberries and mix briefly.
5. Divide dough into small muffin cups, preferably made of silicone. Expect about 2 tbsp batter per muffin. Bake for 25 minutes in the lower part of the oven. Allow to cool.
6. Spread the chocolate cream onto the cakes and top with a small dollop of blueberry and cashew fluff. Optional: decorate with a fresh blueberry.

CHOCOLATE CREAM

4 oz (100 g) chocolate, 70% cocoa

1/2 avocado

2 tbsp honey or agave nectar

DIRECTIONS:

1. Melt chocolate in a double boiler. Let cool and then mix the chocolate with avocado and agave nectar into a smooth paste.

BLUEBERRY AND CASHEW FLUFF

1 cup (100 g) blueberries

1/2 cup (100 ml) cashews

1 tbsp agave nectar or honey

DIRECTIONS:

1. Mix blueberries, nuts, and agave nectar to a creamy consistency.

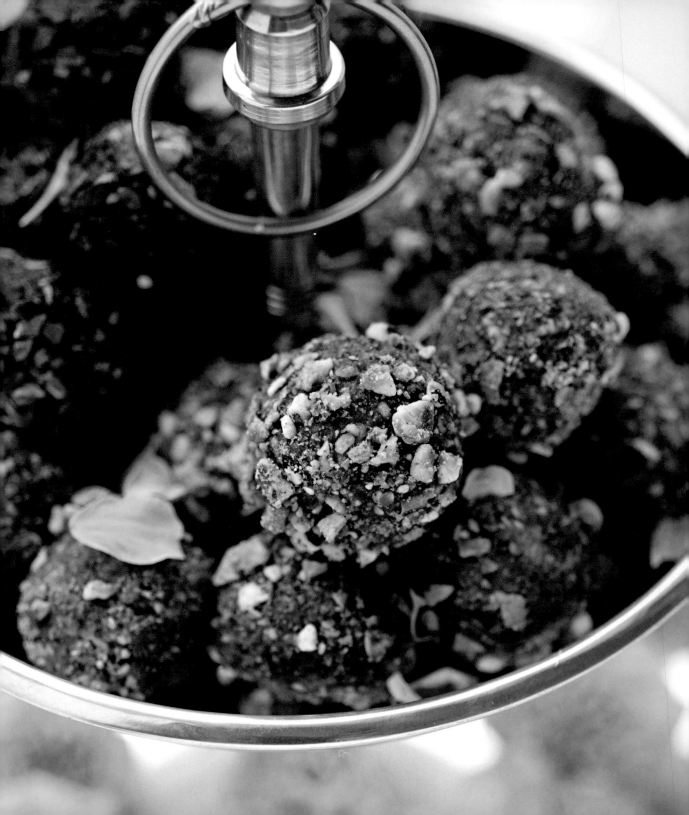

Truffles

Fruit and nut truffles can be made with many possible variations. If the dried fruit is hard, soak it for a few hours. One idea is to put truffle batter into a crust and garnish with fresh fruit and serve with whipped cream.

Apple Truffles

Something so simple and healthy, yet so good.

About 25 balls
1 large apple
1 scant cup (200 ml) raisins
3/4 cup (150 ml) dried dates, soaked 1 hour
3 tsp ground cinnamon
1 tsp ground cardamom
1 scant cup (200 ml) hazelnuts or almonds
1 scant cup (200 ml) cashews
1/4 cup (50 ml) sesame seeds or mixed nuts
   to roll balls in

DIRECTIONS:
1. Grate the apple coarsely and squeeze out most of the liquid. Place raisins, dates, apples, cinnamon, cardamom, and nuts in a food processor.

2. Blend to a coarse mixture. Shape into balls and roll in sesame seeds or nuts that you mixed into a fine powder in a food processor.

Chocolate Balls

Chocolate is always right, whether at the end of a meal or as a mini snack.

About 25 balls
12 dried dates, soaked 1 hour
10 dried apricots
1/2 cup (100 ml) cocoa
seeds of 1 vanilla bean or 1 tsp ground
   vanilla bean
juice of 1/4 lemon
1 1/2 cup (300 ml) cashews
2 tbsp coconut oil
cocoa powder to dust the balls with

DIRECTIONS:
1. Mix dates (pitted), apricots, cocoa, vanilla seeds, and lemon.
2. Add the cashew nuts and coconut oil and blend to a coarse pulp. Shape into balls and dust a little cocoa powder on top.

The picture shows Apple Truffles in front and Chocolate Balls in the upper left.

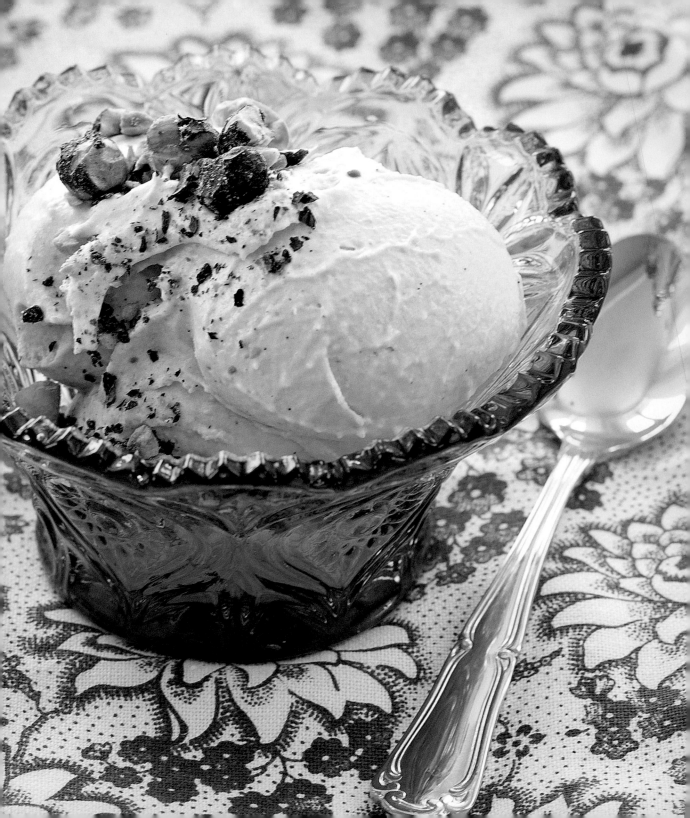

Coconut Ice Cream

Creamy, fresh, and at the same time mild with a fine flavor. Super lovely consistency. You have to try this!

8 servings
2 cups (500 ml) cashews, soaked for 4 hours
1 3/4–2 cups (400–500 ml) coconut milk
1 scant cup (200 ml) agave nectar
1/2 cup (100 ml) coconut
1/4 cup (50 ml) dried coconut
1 vanilla bean
2 pinches sea salt

DIRECTIONS:
1. Place all ingredients in a blender and blend until smooth. Let mixture sit for a while to make it creamy.
2. Cool the mixture and freeze it in an ice cream maker according to the instructions. Serve with fresh fruit and perhaps candied hazelnuts. May be stored in the freezer.

CANDIED HAZELNUTS

Totally perfect for sprinkling over fruit salad or to serve with ice cream.

1 scant cup (200 ml) hazelnuts
1 tbsp maple syrup
1/2 tsp cinnamon

DIRECTIONS:
1. Preheat the oven to 350°F (175°C). Mix the nuts and maple syrup on a baking sheet lined with parchment paper. Dust with cinnamon.
2. Roast for 20 minutes and let cool.
3. If you like, chop coarsely right before serving.

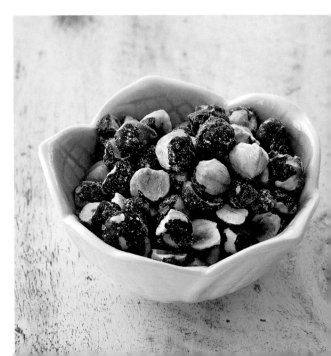

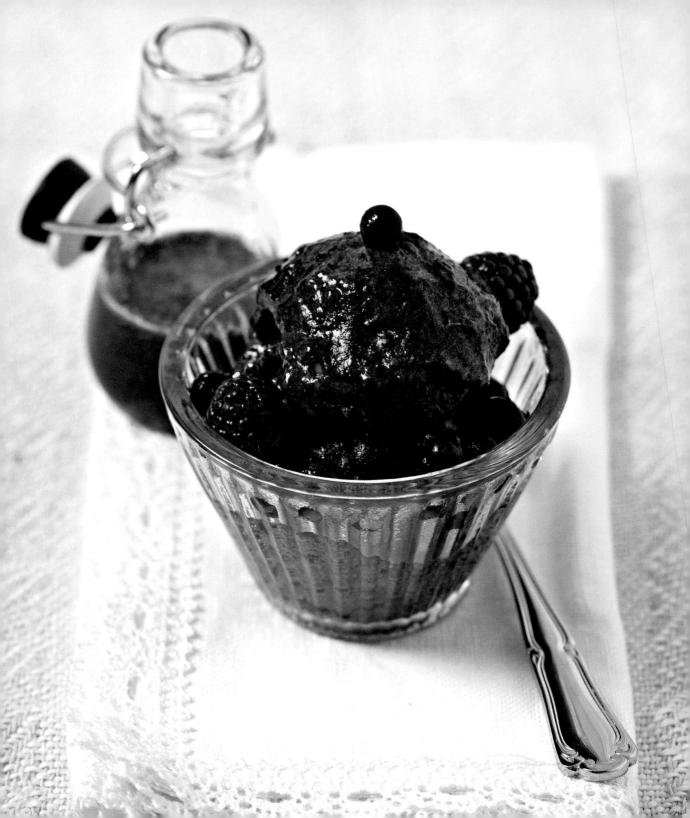

Quick Berry Ice Cream

It's hard to imagine that it could be so easy to make a beautiful and delicious dessert. But it's true!

4 servings
3 frozen bananas
8 oz (225 g) frozen berries
optional: 2 tbsp honey or agave nectar

DIRECTIONS:
1. Mix bananas, cut into pieces, and berries into an ice cream-like batter. Flavor to taste with honey. Eat right away!
2. Serve with basil agave.

BASIL AGAVE
Mix a bunch of basil with 2 tbsp agave nectar to a syrupy consistency.

INDEX